first place
4health

Bible Study Series

the power
of hope

Published by Gospel Light
Ventura, California, U.S.A.
www.gospellight.com
Printed in the U.S.A.

Caution: The information contained in this book is intended to be solely for
informational and educational purposes. It is assumed that the First Place 4 Health
participant will consult a medical or health professional before beginning this or
any other weight-loss or physical fitness program.

Revised and updated from *Renewing Hope*,
published in the First Place Bible Study in 2008.

Library of Congress Cataloging-in-Publication Data
First Place 4 Health Bible study series : the power of hope.
p. cm.
ISBN 978-0-8307-5487-8 (trade paper)
1. Hope—Biblical teaching—Textbooks. 2. Hope—Religious aspects—Christianity—
Textbooks. 3. Weight loss—Religious aspects—Christianity—Textbooks. 4. Health—
Religious aspects—Christianity—Textbooks. I. First Place 4 Health (Organization)
II. Title: Power of hope.
BS680.H7F57 2010
220.8′613712—dc22
2010013197

Rights for publishing this book outside the U.S.A. or in non-English
languages are administered by Gospel Light Worldwide, an international
not-for-profit ministry. For additional information, please visit www.glww.org, email
info@glww.org, or write to Gospel Light Worldwide, 1957 Eastman Avenue, Ventura,
CA 93003, U.S.A.

To order copies of this book and other Gospel Light products in bulk quantities,
please contact us at 1-800-446-7735.

contents

BIBLE STUDIES

ADDITIONAL MATERIALS

foreword

My introduction to Bible study came when I joined First Place in March 1981. I had been attending church since I was a small child, but the extent of my study of the Bible had been reading my Sunday School quarterly on Saturday night. On Sunday morning, I would listen to my Sunday School teacher as she taught God's Word to me. During the worship service, I would listen to our pastor as he taught God's Word to me. Frankly, the idea of digging out the truths of the Bible for myself had never entered my mind.

Perhaps you are right where I was back in 1981. If so, you are in for a blessing you never dreamed possible. As you start studying the truths of the Bible for yourself through the First Place 4 Health Bible studies, you will see God begin to open your understanding of His Word.

Almost every First Place 4 Health member I have talked with about the program says, "The weight loss is wonderful, but the most important thing I have received from my association with First Place 4 Health is learning to study God's Word." The First Place 4 Health Bible studies are designed to be done on a daily basis. As you work through each day's study (which will take 15 to 20 minutes to complete), you will be discovering the deep truths of God's Word. A part of each week's study will also include a Bible memory verse for the week.

There are many in-depth Bible studies on the market. The First Place 4 Health Bible studies are not designed for the purpose of in-depth study, but are designed to be used in conjunction with the rest of the program to bring balance into your life. Our desire is for each member to begin having a personal quiet time with God each day. This time alone with God should include a time of prayer, Bible reading and Bible study. Having a quiet time is a daily discipline that will bring the rich rewards of balance, which is something we all need.

God bless you as you begin this exciting journey toward a balanced life. God will richly bless your efforts to give Him first place in your life. Remember Matthew 6:33: "But seek first his kingdom and his righteousness, and all these things will be given to you as well."

Carole Lewis, First Place 4 Health National Director

introduction

First Place 4 Health is a Christ-centered health program that emphasizes balance in the physical, mental, emotional and spiritual areas of life. The First Place 4 Health program is meant to be a daily process. As we learn to keep Christ first in our lives, we will find that He is the One who satisfies our hunger and our every need.

This Bible study is designed to be used in conjunction with the First Place 4 Health program but can be beneficial for anyone interested in obtaining a balanced lifestyle. The Bible study has been created in a five-day format, with the last two days reserved for reflection on the material studied. Keep in mind that the ultimate goal of studying the Bible is not only for knowledge but also for application and a changed life. Don't feel anxious if you can't seem to find the *correct* answer. Many times, the Word will speak differently to different people, depending on where they are in their walk with God and the season of life they are experiencing. Be prepared to discuss with your fellow First Place 4 Health members what you learned that week through your study.

There are some additional components included with this study that will be helpful as you pursue the goal of giving Christ first place in every area of your life:

- **Group Prayer Request Form:** This form is at the end of each week's study. You can use this to record any special requests that might be given in class.

- **Leader Discussion Guide:** This discussion guide is provided to help the First Place 4 Health leader guide a group through this Bible study. It includes ideas for facilitating a First Place 4 Health class discussion for each week of the Bible study.

- **Two Weeks of Menu Plans with Recipes:** There are 14 days of meals, and all are interchangeable. Each day totals 1,400 to 1,500 calories and includes snacks. Instructions are given for those who need more calories. An accompanying grocery list includes items needed for each week of meals.

- **First Place 4 Health Member Survey:** Fill this out and bring it to your first meeting. This information will help your leader know your interests and talents.

- **Personal Weight and Measurement Record:** Use this form to keep a record of your weight loss. Record any loss or gain on the chart after the weigh-in at each week's meeting.

- **Weekly Prayer Partner Forms:** Fill out this form before class and place it into a basket during the class meeting. After class, you will draw out a prayer request form, and this will be your prayer partner for the week. Try to call or email the person sometime before the next class meeting to encourage that person.

- **Live It Trackers:** Your Live It Tracker is to be completed at home and turned in to your leader at your weekly First Place 4 Health meeting. The Tracker is designed to help you practice mindfulness and stay accountable with regard to your eating and exercise habits. Step-by-step instructions for how to use the Live It Tracker are provided in the *Member's Guide*.

- **Let's Count Our Miles!** A worthy goal we encourage is for you to complete 100 miles of exercise during your 12 weeks in First Place 4 Health. There are many activities listed on pages 255-256 that count toward your goal of 100 miles. When you complete a mile of activity, mark off the box listed on the Hundred Mile Club chart located on the inside of the back cover.

- **Scripture Memory Cards:** These cards have been designed so you can use them while exercising. It is suggested that you punch a hole in the upper left corner and place the cards on a ring. You may want to take the cards in the car or to work so you can practice each week's Scripture memory verse throughout the day.

- **Scripture Memory CD:** All 10 Scripture memory verses have been put to music at an exercise tempo in the CD at the back of this study. Use this CD when exercising or even when you are just driving in your car. The words of Scripture are often easier to memorize when accompanied by music.

welcome to
The Power of Hope

At your first group meeting for this session of First Place 4 Health, you will meet your fellow members, get an overview of your materials and find out what you can expect at weekly meetings. The majority of your class time will be spent learning about the four-sided person concept, the Live It Food Plan, and how change begins from the inside out. You will also have a chance to ask any questions about how to get the most out of First Place 4 Health. If possible, complete the Member Survey on page 205 before your first group meeting. The information that you give will help your leader tailor the next 12 weeks to the needs of the whole group.

Each weekly meeting begins with a weigh-in for members. This will allow you to track your progress over the 12-week session. Your Week One weigh-in/measurement will establish a baseline of comparison so that you can set healthy goals for this session. If you are apprehensive about weighing in every week, talk with your group leader about your concerns. He or she will have some options for you to consider that will make the weigh-in activity encouraging rather than stressful.

The day after your first meeting, begin Week Two of this Bible study. This session, you and your group will recognize areas of your life that are out of balance and learn God's way of regaining your equilibrium. As you open yourself to the truth of Scripture and share your hopes and struggles with the members of your group during the next 12 weeks, you'll find yourself becoming the healthy child of God you are designed to be!

heartsick and battle weary

SCRIPTURE MEMORY VERSE
Hope deferred makes the heart sick,
But a longing fulfilled is a tree of life.
PROVERBS 13:12

This proverb tells it all: facing a failure when we are seeking to achieve a weight loss or fitness goal can lead us to feeling heartsick and battle weary. Perhaps we began a new weight-loss program with high hopes and grand dreams, and in the beginning we might have even seen noticeable results. Our spirits soared as the pounds and inches seemed to melt away. Yet for many of us this was only a temporary success, and we gained back the pounds we lost—plus a few more. By the time many of us come to First Place 4 Health we are fairly certain of what *doesn't* work, but we aren't sure that a balanced program based on proven biblical principles will work either. We've lost our enthusiasm, our motivation, our dignity and, in the end, the most important thing of all: our *hope.*

But as hopeless as the prospect of achieving lifelong fitness and health may seem, we should take heart. All positive change begins with awareness—with an honest admission that the way we have done things in the past doesn't work. As this week's memory verse so poignantly reminds us, a longing fulfilled is a tree of life. But in order to achieve a life of health, wholeness and balance, we must first be honest with ourselves about (1) our present condition, and (2) the futility of past efforts not based on seeking Christ first, no matter how well intentioned those efforts might have been.

As you begin this study, spend a few moments reflecting on where you are, where you hope to be, and what has kept you from reaching your health and fitness goals in the past. Remember, fearless honesty is the gateway to hope, so be truthful in your assessment. Falling into denial will only prolong the deferred hope that is keeping your heart sick and your body weary.

CRUEL TASKMASTERS

Loving and compassionate Lord, I confess any time I have not treated myself well. Today I ask You to help me realize the precious child of God that I am.

Not taking proper care of our bodies is a form of self-imposed oppression in which we become our own cruel taskmasters. Fortunately, we can learn how to break the chains that keep us bound in this destructive cycle by observing another oppressed people: the children of Israel under the tyranny of Pharaoh and the ruthless Egyptian slave drivers. Turn in your Bible to Exodus 1 and read verses 1-14 to get an overview of what had happened to God's Chosen People. What was the Israelites' situation?

placed in bondage

Look up the word "ruthless" in a dictionary, which is the word used in verses 13 and 14 to describe the Egyptian taskmasters. Write the meaning of this word in the space below.

without mercy or pity

Verse 14 tells us that the ruthless way in which the Israelites were treated made their lives bitter. Have you had past feelings that made your life seem bitter? If so, describe some of these feelings below.

Feeling jealous - unloved or values

Even though the Israelites were under cruel oppression, they were not without hope. Read Exodus 3:7. What action did they take—which was the only real action that they could take given their circumstances?

Cried out to God

According to Exodus 3:7, God heard their cries. What emotion did those cries produce in Him over the plight of His chosen ones?

take action (concern) about the suffering

Do you believe that if you cry out to God, He will see, hear and be concerned about you? Why or why not?

yes

If you are feeling distressed, spend some time today crying out to God, confident that He is concerned with your plight and will send a "Moses" to deliver you.

God, I thank You that You are the One who sees my plight, hears my misery, is concerned for my wellbeing and comes to my assistance. Amen.

CRIES OF DELIVERANCE

Day 2

O Lord God Almighty, I will give You thanks, for You are good and Your love for me endures forever (see Psalm 107:1).

Psalm 107 is an epic-style description of God's goodness and enduring love. Turn to that psalm now. How are God's people described in verse 2?

redeemed

From what have God's people been redeemed?

Slavery - enemy - oppression - poverty

There are four groups of people in perilous situations described in this psalm. The first group is found in Psalm 107:4-5. What was the situation these people faced?

Lost : confusion hungry thirsty but No Life

According to Psalm 107:6, what did these hungry and thirsty people do?

Cried out to the Lord

What did God do in response to their cries (see vv. 6-7)?

Delivered them from their distress

What does the psalmist tell us we should do when we experience God's unfailing love (see v. 8)?

give thanks

What assurance of God's goodness do the words of Psalm 107:9 provide?

It brings a satisfaction to your life

Those of us who have traveled through the "Desert of Diet Horrors" know what it is like to be hungry and thirsty. What hope can you glean from today's lesson?

God can and will help if we let Him.

God cares, my choices matter to Him

Lord, in Your goodness You have redeemed me from the hand of the foe. You promise to satisfy the thirsty and fill the hungry with good things. How blessed I am that You are the God who cares for me (see Psalm 107:2).

DARKNESS AND GLOOM

Day **3**

Compassionate and merciful Father, forgive me for those times I have rebelled against Your words and not listened to Your wise counsel (see Psalm 107:11). Help me to listen to Your voice today. Amen.

Yesterday we studied Psalm 107, and today we will continue to look at this account of God's goodness and love. The second group of distressed people are found in Psalm 107:10-12. Read those verses and summarize the trouble in which those people found themselves.

According to verse 11, why had this misfortune come upon them?

In our modern vernacular, what word or words would we use for "darkness and gloom"?

Depression and despair keep us imprisoned in darkness and gloom more securely than the iron chains described in Psalm 107. How might depression and despair have been part of your plight in the past?

_____

_____

_____

_____

_____

Psalm 107:13 tells us about a specific action the people sitting in darkness and gloom took. What was that action?

_____

_____

_____

_____

As a result of their cries, what action did the Lord take on their behalf (see v. 14)?

_____

_____

_____

_____

What is the proper response of those who have been freed from the chains that kept them in darkness and gloom (see v. 15)?

_____

_____

_____

_____

Unlike the children of Israel we learned about in our Day 1 study, these people were not the victims of cruel slavery. Their misery was the result of bad choices. Yet God still came to their rescue when they cried out to Him. What does that tell you about the mercy and compassion of God?

_____

_____

_____

_____

Spend some time thanking God for breaking the chains that keep people in darkness, gloom, depression and despair.

O Lord God, You have set me free from my prison, and I will
praise Your holy name (see Psalm 142:7).

GOD'S SAVING WORD — Day 4

O Lord Most High, thank You for sending Your Word to heal me. You have,
indeed, been good to me. Today I will sing Your praise. Amen.

As we continue our study of Psalm 107, spend a few moments thinking about what we have studied so far this week about crying out to God. Now read Psalm 107:17-18, which describes the third group of people in calamity. After reading these verses, write a brief summary of their situation in the space below.

_____

_____

_____

_____

How did these people respond to the calamity, and how did their action bring relief (see v. 19)?

_____

_____

_____

_____

During our Day 2 and Day 3 studies, we have seen God satisfying hunger and thirst and breaking bonds of depression and despair. Psalm 107:20 gives us a specific action God took to heal the people who had suffered great affliction. What was that action?

_____

_____

_____

_____

_____

God has also sent forth His Word to heal and rescue us! How can reading the Bible, studying Scripture and committing God's Word to memory be part of our deliverance?

_____

_____

_____

_____

In light of Psalm 107:20, why must any effort we take to be free of unhealthy habits or bondage to food be based on God's Word?

_____

_____

_____

_____

Psalm 107:21-22 once again outlines the proper response of those who have been rescued from a life of misery. What are the elements of thanksgiving and praise that we find in these verses?

_____

_____

_____

_____

What song of joy can you sing to the Lord today that will tell of God's goodness to you? Do so now!

Thank You, gracious God, for allowing me to tell others of Your goodness and grace as I become a living witness of the healing power of Your mighty Word. Amen.

SAFE HAVEN

Day 5

O Lord, You are the One who calms the storms of my life and brings me to a safe harbor. I would be lost without Your love. Thank You, Lord. Amen.

This week, we have been looking at the benefits of recognizing our plight and feelings of hopelessness and crying out to God in our distress. What does crying out to God have to do with the honest assessment you were asked to make of your present situation at the beginning of this study?

_____

_____

_____

_____

_____

Our final group of people in peril is found in Psalm 107:23-27. Read these verses carefully and describe why these merchants were at their wits' end.

_____

_____

_____

_____

_____

Unlike some of the other people we have seen in distress this week, these people were not in danger because of their own rebellion and iniquity, nor were they the victims of the cruel action of others. There is no foe mentioned. What has caused their distress?

_____

_____

_____

_____

Like those caught in the storm at sea, we are often left reeling and staggering by circumstances beyond our control. Are you dealing with a situation that you feel powerless to change? If so, describe that situation.

_____

_____

_____

_____

How has this situation brought you to your wit's end?

_____

_____

_____

_____

Even though we are all powerless in our human understanding and effort, who is available to help us in our distress (see Psalm 107:28)?

_____

_____

_____

_____

According to Psalm 107:29, what did God do to the roaring sea and raging storm?

_____

_____

_____

_____

What does Psalm 107:28-29 tell us about the importance of prayer when we find ourselves in danger?

_____

_____

_____

_____

Psalm 107:30 tells us that as a result of the cries of those whose courage had melted away, God took a specific action. What was that action, and what emotion did it evoke in the people?

_____

_____

_____

_____

Once again, Psalm 107:31-32 shows us the proper response to God's goodness. Verse 32 even gives us two specific places where we are to express our gratitude. What are those two places, and how might telling your First Place 4 Health group about the good things God has done for you be part of what is being described in this verse?

_____

_____

_____

_____

End today's study by spending some time journaling about God's incredible goodness to you, especially as it applies to the safe haven He has provided for you when you cry out to Him for help.

Gracious Father, Your love is unfailing and Your deeds are wonderful.
Thank You for showering me with goodness and kindness. Amen.

REFLECTION AND APPLICATION

*Lord God, even though years of deferred hope may have made my heart sick,
I will trust You to fulfill the longing of my heart (see Proverbs 13:12). Amen.*

This week, we have looked at some of the things that may defer our hope. Reflecting back on this week's study, why is making honest assessment of your situation a prelude to having your hope renewed? In other words, what does that honest assessment allow you to do, and why is this action a vital part of the renewal process?

_____

_____

_____

_____

_____

This week's memory verse refers to a "tree of life." What does that expression tell you about your life here on earth? (In giving your answer, think about the life cycle of a tree, from the time the seed falls into the fertile ground until the inner rings that reveal the events that have taken place during the tree's lifetime are visible.)

_____

_____

_____

_____

How might some of the events described in Psalm 107:4-32 be part of the inner rings that tell the story of your life's journey?

_____

_____

_____

_____

After studying the lives of people in distress during this week's study, what new behavior(s) have you learned that you can put into place to begin renewing the hope within you?

_____

_____

_____

_____

What is keeping you from doing those things right now?

_____

_____

_____

_____

Lord, You have redeemed me from every foe, and today I recall Your goodness and grace. When I was at my wit's end, You heard my cries and came to my assistance. I will praise You in the assembly; I will tell others of Your unfailing love (see Psalm 107:32).

REFLECTION AND APPLICATION

Day 7

O Lord, You see my distress, hear my cries and are concerned for my wellbeing. Thank You for Your goodness, grace and unfailing love.

Much of this week's study has been taken from Psalm 107. We have seen people in distress—distress that was the result of many different things. Which of the four groups of people we have looked at in Psalm 107 can you most closely identify with? Why?

_____

_____

_____

_____

During this week's lessons, we have examined many truths that reinforce God's goodness, grace and unfailing love. Pause for a moment and recall something new you learned about God from this week's study. Describe that in the space below.

_____

_____

_____

_____

Now read Psalm 107:33-43. Just as the first 32 verses in this psalm teach us about God's grace, compassion and unfailing love, these last 10 verses teach us about another attribute of the God we worship and serve. What did you learn about God from reading these verses?

_____

_____

_____

Why do you think the psalmist declares, "The upright see and rejoice, but all the wicked shut their mouths," in Psalm 107:42?

_____

_____

_____

Psalm 107 ends with the words, "Whoever is wise, let him heed these things and consider the great love of the Lord" (v. 43). What admonition found in Psalm 107 do you need to heed?

_____

_____

_____

Today, spend time considering the great love of the Lord. You might want to record your thoughts in a journal. In your writing, praise God that He has allowed you to be part of His Chosen People, those who see and rejoice in the great things that He has done for the undeserving recipients of His unfathomable grace.

O God of hope, I pray that You will fill me with peace and joy as I trust in You so that I will soon be overflowing with hope by the power of the Holy Spirit (see Romans 15:13). Today, Sovereign Lord, I will be among the wise that heed Your Word and consider the great love of the Lord (see Psalm 107:43).

Group Prayer Requests

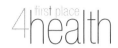

Today's Date: _____

Name	Request

Results

_____

_____

_____

_____

_____

put your hope in God

SCRIPTURE MEMORY VERSE

Why are you downcast, O my soul? Why so disturbed within me?
Put your hope in God, for I will yet praise him, my Savior and my God.

PSALM 42:5-6

When we think of the word "downcast," we usually think of it as synonymous with being discouraged or depressed. However, the Hebrew word translated as "downcast" in this passage (*shachach*) can also refer to being "bowed down" or "weakened." We see this usage in Psalm 38:6, where the psalmist David writes, "I am bowed down and brought very low; all day long I go about mourning." David felt "downcast" and "weakened" because of the realization of his sin before God. His soul was troubled, and the only way out was for him to confess his sin and put his hope in God.

David often felt downcast in his soul. For years he was pursued by King Saul and forced to live like a fugitive, even though he had been anointed as Israel's next king. Later, David's own son, Absalom, threatened David's reign, and once again the great king was forced to hide in caves rather than enjoy the comforts of his palace. Of course, sometimes David brought these situations on himself, such as when he committed adultery with Bathsheba (see 2 Samuel 11). After Nathan the prophet confronted him with his sin, David wrote, "I know my transgressions, and my sin is always before me. . . . Create in me a pure heart, O God, and renew a steadfast spirit within me" (Ps. 51:3,10).

This week, we will take a closer look at how we, like David, can put our hope in God when our soul is feeling downcast and we need to rely on the strength of the Lord to pull us through.

Day 1

THE GOOD SHEPHERD

O Lord God, I am so grateful that You are the Good Shepherd, the One who hears even my faintest cry and rescues me from the lion's mouth. Amen.

The first time we are introduced to the story of David in the Bible is in 1 Samuel 16. Read 1 Samuel 16:10-12. What was David doing when Samuel paid his father, Jesse, a visit to anoint one of his sons to be the next king of Israel?

tending Sheep

Turn to Psalm 23 and read David's hymn of praise to the Lord. Ezekiel 34:31 gives insight into why David wrote the psalm the way he did. What thoughts and emotions come up for you as you contemplate the Shepherd's role in your life?

God is Good, Loving, my Friend

In 1 Samuel 17:34-37, David describes some specific action he took on behalf of the sheep entrusted to his care. What did David do when predators threatened the safety of the flock? What does this Scripture passage tell you about the flock?

rescued it
He will rescue us from every hard space, and distroy the enemy

Now turn to 1 Peter 5:8. Who does the lion in David's story represent?

Lies

How might God be using what you are learning in this study and through the tools provided in the First Place 4 Health program to rescue you from the lion's mouth?

Self worth, self confidence

How would David know when a predator was carrying off one of the sheep from his flock?

_Cry out...
He Know all + every one
Doesn't miss a thing_

What does the rescue of one sheep from a large flock tell you about God, our Good Shepherd and the chief overseer of our souls?

I matter...

How does knowing that you are a sheep in the Good Shepherd's care give you renewed hope?

There help for me,

Watchful and caring Shepherd, I know Satan roams around like a roaring lion hunting for prey. Thank You for keeping watch over me. Amen.

DOWNCAST SHEEP

Gracious Lord, You are the overseer and shepherd of my soul. Thank You that I am kept safe in the palm of Your mighty, outstretched hand. Amen.

Phillip Keller, a lay pastor in Northern Africa, was a shepherd by trade. From his experience herding sheep, he wrote a book titled *A Shepherd Looks at the 23rd Psalm*. In this book, Keller writes a description of what the word "downcast," as used in this week's memory verse, means:

> This is an old English shepherd's term for a sheep that has turned over on its back and cannot get up again by itself. A "cast" sheep is a very pathetic sight. Lying on its back, its feet in the air, it flails away frantically struggling to stand up, without success. Sometimes it will bleat a little for help, but generally it lies there lashing about in frightened frustration. If the owner does not arrive on the scene within a reasonably short time, the sheep will die. This is but another reason why it is so essential for a careful sheepman to look over his flock every day, counting them to see that all are able to be up and on their feet. It is not only the shepherd who keeps a sharp eye for cast sheep, but also the predators. Buzzards, vultures, dogs, coyotes and cougars all know that a cast sheep is easy prey and death is not far off. This knowledge that any "cast" sheep is helpless, close to death and vulnerable to attack, makes the whole problem of cast sheep serious for the manager.[1]

Now turn to Psalm 139:1-6 and read these verses. In light of Phillip Keller's description of a "cast sheep," what words in Psalm 139:1-6 give you hope and comfort? Explain your answer by using words directly from this psalm.

He knows me, you perceive my thoughts, you r familiar with my ways, your hand is upon me

Psalm 139:6 describes this knowledge as "too _Wonderful_ for me, too _Lofty_ for me to attain." What feelings and thoughts come up when you consider the truth that God is always with you—that He sees everything you do and knows every thought you think?

Safe Loved, cared for, desired Interest, facinated with

How might your efforts to take care of yourself change if you realized this truth at a heart level rather than only as head knowledge?

Hopeful matter

In our memory verse for this week, the psalmist says that his soul is downcast. Using Phillip Keller's description of a cast sheep, what valuable information can we learn about a downcast soul?

it can die if it does get up right Struggle without success Frustrated, Frightened

What is the downcast soul's fate if help does not arrive soon? Who is the only one who can right a downcast soul?

Death, Jesus

Who besides the Good Shepherd notices that the sheep is downcast?

prediators Buzzards Vultures, dogs cayotes + cougars

What does this tell you about the importance of the spiritual component in your health journey?

It is not just a natural battle
But a spiritual battle.

Your love, O God, is too wonderful for me to comprehend. Although I don't fully understand Your grace, I am thankful that I am a sheep in Your care.

Day 3

THE LOST

Lord, when I was still a sinner, Christ died for me! Thank You for being the Good Shepherd who laid down His life so I might spend eternity with You.

In fulfillment of the Scriptures, Jesus Christ came to save His people from their sins. In John 10, Jesus describes Himself using specific terminology. Turn to John 10:11 and write that truth below:

Laid down his Life for me

Now read John 10:14-15. What else do we learn about the Good Shepherd in these verses?

Jesus is the good shephard + He knows me + I know Him
Papa knows Jesus Laid down His Life for me

Isaiah 53:6 gives us another truth about the Good Shepherd's flock. What does Isaiah tell us?

We all have gone astray, but the Lord has take on our weaknesses

How is that truth borne out in Romans 5:8?

He did it because He love us

He traded our death for His

Recall our lessons from Week Two. There was a different reason that each of the four groups of people found themselves in great danger. What were those reasons?

Group One (see Psalm 107:4-5)

Lost: trying to find satifaction
in things that don't give life

Group Two (see Psalm 107:10-11)

Rebellion   Oppression
It sin to not follow the councel
of the Lord

Group Three (see Psalm 107:17-18)

Foolish Rebellion
opposed the Live giver
Draw near to death

Group Four (see Psalm 107:23-27)

Fearful- runners

When these people cried out to the Lord, did the reason for their affliction influence His response? What was his reaction to their cries? Write
the phrase in the space below that describes what God did (see vv.
6,13,19,20,28).

He lead by a straight way to settle
He saved them from their distress
Sent out His word + healed them
rescued them from the grave

How will this direct you the next time you find yourself "downcast"?

Know God is the redeemer
Not try to help myself
Look to him

In Luke 19:10, Jesus gives us His "mission statement." Write those words
in the space below.

For the son of Man came to seek
and to save the Lost

How does Luke 19:10 verify the truth that the Good Shepherd saves the
downcast sheep?

He came to seek, Look for +
Rescue

What would you like to say to Jesus, your Good Shepherd, after completing today's study?

*Lord God Almighty, You are my Good Shepherd. I have heard Your
voice and I will follow You. Amen.*

HOPE IN GOD

Heavenly Father, as the deer pants for streams of water, so today my soul pants for You, O God (see Psalm 42:1).

Take a few moments to contemplate this week's memory verse. If you were to ask your soul the question, "Why are you downcast, why so disturbed within me?" what would be your soul's answer?

I don't KNOW ...

Look at the first four verses of Psalm 42. How does the psalmist describe his soul-condition in verses 1-2?

hunger, desperation, confusion

What does it mean to have a soul that is thirsty—a soul that is panting for God?

Desperate, needy, humble

What did the psalmist do in the past that he is not able to do now, and how is this a contributing factor in the dry, thirsty condition of his soul (see v. 4)?

Praise God, be thankful

Most Bible scholars agree that when this psalm was written, the people had either been under attack from the Aramean king Hazael (about 800 B.C.; see 2 Kings 12:17-18) or from the Babylonians, who destroyed Jerusalem and the Temple in 587 B.C. (see 2 Kings 25). They could no longer go to the Temple and worship God in the company of God's people. How does the psalmist describe the experience of leading God's people to the house of God in verse 4?

I used to go with the multitude, leading the _____ to the house of God , with voice of joy and praise among the festive throng.

What does this verse tell you about the importance of being part of a body of believers who worship the Lord with joy and thanksgiving?

there is hope + power to unity

How might your First Place 4 Health group also be part of the throng that nourishes your soul when it is weary?

encourage, support, focus, hope

Unlike the people of Israel, we do not need to go to a specific place to worship. God, in the person of the Holy Spirit, dwells in our hearts through faith in Jesus Christ, our Lord. What would you like to say right now in praise to God?

Thank You, loving Lord, that I can be part of a First Place 4 Health group that worships You with shouts of joy and thanksgiving. Amen.

REMEMBERING GOD'S GOODNESS

Lord, today I will demolish every thought that is contrary to Your Word. I will make a positive attitude part of my renewed hope (see 2 Corinthians 10:5).

After asking his soul a question, what does the psalmist tell himself to do in the words of this week's memory verse (see v. 5)?

demolish every thought contrary to truth.
make a positive attitude part of may renewed hope

What does the way the psalmist talks to himself tell you about the importance of maintaining a healthy and positive attitude at all times? How can this be part of your First Place 4 Health program?

stay fowsed ,up Lifted
embrace God Love + truths of
myself take captive

According to 2 Corinthians 10:5, what are we to do with every thought that is contrary to the Word of God?

Demolish arguments and every
pretension that sets itself up
against the knowledge of God

What is the psalmist's vow at the end of Psalm 42:5?

Put your Hope in God
For I will yet praise Him, my
Savior, my God

In response to that vow, what did the psalmist do next (see vv. 6-8)?

prayed

Psalm 77 also affirms the importance of how we view God. Read the entire psalm and describe from verses 10-12 the overarching principle.

remember - meditate on the
Goodness of God

How might keeping a journal of your thoughts and prayers about daily events connect to the psalmist's vow in verse 11?

helps to remember - gives hope
see the hand of God

How is remembering God's past actions part of renewing your hope?

You see God present activity in
every day moments

Admitting that you are in distress, crying out to God for assistance and then putting your hope in Him is the beginning of a process that turns deferred hope into expectant hope. How would you describe the renewing of your hope today?

I walking to a desire I believe
Papa put in me

Gracious Father, thank You for Your faithfulness and love, a love that is not dependent on my feelings or actions, my moods or my accomplishments.

REFLECTION AND APPLICATION

*Thank You, gracious and loving Lord, for the great and precious promises
that You give to me to remind me of Your constant presence
in my life and Your everlasting love. Amen.*

Although your soul may not be downcast right now, most of us know all too well what it is like to be depressed. In Psalm 42, the psalmist described it as a thirsty soul; others speak of it as spiritual dryness or the dark night of the soul.

Although we know what depression feels like, what we often fail to realize is that depression signals the need for us to take immediate action. It is not a time to fall back in defeat, but rather a time for us to take decisive action—to run swiftly to the Word of God. We cannot wait until we feel like reading Scripture and praying. Our feelings are part of the funk we are in. When we find our spiritual strength failing, we need an immediate transfusion of hope and power—whether or not we feel like getting that infusion. We need to pick up our Bible, open it to passages that contain promises of strength and provision and read the words *out loud*.

We need to force-feed our hearts and minds and be encouraged by listening to ourselves recite the words that will renew our strength— the words that God will use to minister to our need. Although force-feeding is a concept that seems to run contrary to the principles of First Place 4 Health, when we're talking about feeding on the Word of God and crying out to the Source of our strength in prayer, we will find help to not lose heart.

There is no need to give in to feelings of discouragement and depression when we have His Word and His great promises to sustain us. Those who trust in Him are never disappointed.

*Almighty God, when feelings of depression set in and I am in danger
of slipping into despondency and despair, I will meditate on Your love
and kindness and draw my strength from Your Word. Amen.*

Day
7

REFLECTION AND APPLICATION

O Lord God, today I will dare to ask myself, "Why are you downcast, O my soul?" and then I will begin to praise You with music and song, confident that I can put my hope in You because You are my Savior and my God.

Somewhere between 1527 and 1529, Martin Luther penned the words of the time-honored hymn "A Mighty Fortress Is Our God," which is a paraphrase of Psalm 46. The first line of that beautiful hymn reads, "A mighty fortress is our God, a bulwark never failing."[2] Not the kind of words we would expect to come from a man who suffered from depression.

Although we are inclined to think of Martin Luther as a giant of the faith, in his lifetime, Martin Luther suffered from many problems—mental and physical—just as we do. As a result of his personal experience, he searched the Scriptures for a remedy for his depression and found that the Divine Physician had just the right prescription to replace his inner gloom with joy and gladness.

We can also benefit from the Divine Physician's remedy when we find ourselves in times of darkness and despair. The Lord sent His Word to heal us. Here are some ways that you can avail yourself of God's grace when you find your soul downcast:

- Music. King Saul was soothed when David played the harp. Paul and Silas sang when imprisoned and chained in the dungeon. Scripture tells us that music makes our heart glad. It is difficult to be depressed when singing songs of praise and thanksgiving to God!

- Praise. All the saints, in every age, agree on this depression remedy. When we can't feel God's presence—or even focus our thoughts enough to pray—we can thank God for the simple blessings of His creation.

- God's Word. God can (and does) use any portion of Scripture to minister to us during times of depression; but throughout the centuries God's people have used the psalms as an anchor when the dark clouds of depression appeared on the horizon.

- God's Spirit. Jesus, just before His crucifixion, comforted His grieving disciples by assuring them of the Spirit's presence. He longs to impart that same comfort to you too.

- God's promises. Gloom gives way to joy when we remember what God has done for us in the past and what He promises to give us in the future. Begin to recall the way God has been your help in the past, confident that He is the same yesterday, today and forever.

Part of a balanced life is learning how to deal with depression in healthy, life-affirming ways. But all too often we self-medicate with excess food, excess spending, excess activity. These things in excess become part of the problem, not the solution. If today you find yourself with a downcast soul, try these simple remedies—listening to and singing music that glorifies God, speaking God's praises, reading God's Word, drawing near to God's Spirit, trusting in God's promises. Like the psalmist—and Martin Luther—you can put your hope in God and praise Him, for He is your Savior and your God.

Forgive me, merciful Father, for those times I do not avail myself of the means of Your grace, choosing instead to wallow in feelings of self-pity and depression. Sovereign Lord, You are my only hope. Today I will put my confidence in You, trusting that when I do so, I will not be disappointed. Amen.

Notes
1. W. Phillip Keller, *A Shepherd Looks at the 23rd Psalm* (Grand Rapids, MI: Zondervan, 1996), pp. 52-53.
2. "A Mighty Fortress Is Our God," *Hymns for the Family of God* (Nashville, TN: Paragon Associates, Inc., 1976), p. 118.

Group Prayer Requests

4 first place health

Today's Date: _____

Name	Request

Results

forgiveness renews hope

Scripture Memory Verse
He has rescued us from the dominion of darkness and brought us into the kingdom of the Son he loves, in whom we have redemption, the forgiveness of sins.
Colossians 1:13-14

For the past two weeks, we have looked at a problem that our memory verse for Week One described as *deferred hope*. According to that verse, deferred hope has a profound effect on our wellbeing. What fruit does deferred hope produce?

What does Proverbs 13:12 tell us brings renewed hope?

Why do you think the writer of this proverb would equate renewed hope to a tree of life?

There are two inner attitudes that stunt the growth of this life-giving tree faster than any outside forces:

1. Guilt over things we have done
2. Bitterness over the things that have been done to us

For hope to flourish into a fruit-producing, life-sustaining tree, we must eliminate these two toxic conditions.

Day 1 — DEALING WITH DENIAL

Compassionate Father, forgive me for any times I try to whitewash my sin rather than coming to You with a broken and contrite heart. Amen.

It has been said that the role of a prophet is to comfort the afflicted and afflict the comfortable. Throughout the Old Testament we see God's prophets bringing consolation to those who are downtrodden and op-pressed—and proclaiming the need for repentance to those who persist in their sin. One of the problems God's true prophets continually dealt with were false prophets who tried to assuage the guilt of the people by whitewashing sin.

Turn to Jeremiah 8:4-12. In your own words, write what God is saying through the prophet Jeremiah.

_____

_____

_____

_____

According to Jeremiah 8:6, what is happening because the people are not asking the question, "What have I done?"

_____

_____

_____

_____

What does God say the prophets and priests are practicing when they do not call sin, sin (see v. 10)?

_____

_____

_____

_____

_____

Jeremiah 8:11 goes so far as to say that these deceitful teachers are dressing the wounds of God's people lightly. They are saying _____, _____ when there is no _____. Stop for a moment and think about an emergency medical technician putting a small bandage on a deep, gaping wound. What would happen if a serious injury were treated like a minor scrape?

_____

_____

_____

_____

Think back to the downcast sheep from last week's study. What would have happened had the shepherd denied that the sheep was in danger?

_____

_____

_____

_____

How is ignoring emotional and spiritual wellbeing, and attending only to the physical side of health, like putting a Band-Aid on a gaping wound?

_____

_____

_____

_____

How might you be denying the existence of a life-threatening condition when you carry around guilt and bitterness?

_____

_____

_____

_____

> *Thank You, Lord, for sending Your prophetic Word to comfort me in my affliction, and afflict me when I am comfortable in my sin.*

Day 2

THE PRICE OF PEACE

Lord, help me not to settle for the world's peace. Help me truly realize in the depth of my soul that only faith in Jesus Christ can bring me lasting peace.

While false prophets throughout the ages have tried to convince us that peace without sacrifice is possible, God's infallible Word tells a much different story! Turn to Isaiah 53, the words of another prophet, and read God's version of the price of peace. This passage is a foretelling of Jesus Christ's sacrificial death on the cross so that we can be at peace with God. According to Isaiah 53:4-5, Jesus, the Lamb of God, carried four things to Calvary's cross. List them below:

1. _____

2. _____

3. _____

4. _____

What type of infirmities or maladies did Jesus carry for us? Because this passage is about peace with God, how would you describe the sorrows Jesus bore on the cross?

_____

_____

_____

_____

Do you think those sorrows also include the sadness we feel when going through grief, loss or depression? Explain your answer.

_____

_____

_____

_____

_____

_____

Write the words of Isaiah 53:5 below, letting them sink into your soul even as you put them down on paper:

But he was _____ for our _____, he was crushed
for our _____; the _____ that brought us
_____ was _____ him, and by his _____ we
are _____.

Isaiah 53 ends with a bold declaration. Write the last sentence of verse 12 in the space below.

_____

_____

_____

_____

_____

Spend some time today thanking Jesus for coming to earth in human form to be the atoning sacrifice for your sin. If you are not sure that you are among those for whom Christ died, talk to a pastor, spiritual director or Christian friend to find out how you, too, can call Jesus Christ your Lord and Savior.

> *Gentle Shepherd, You came to lay down Your life for Your sheep. Thank You that I am among the flock for whom You died (see John 10:15). Amen.*

Day 3 CONFESSING TRANSGRESSIONS

My Lord and my God, thank You for calling me out of darkness into Your marvelous light. Amen.

The apostle John, "the beloved disciple," wrote some words that can help us understand the importance of confession. Read 1 John 1:5-10 to discover what he told the flock of believers under his care about sin. (Keep your Bible open to this passage, as we will be discussing a number of points from this text.)

From whom did the apostle John hear the message referred to in verse 5 (see vv. 3-4)? What action words tell you John was up close and personal with the message?

_____

_____

_____

_____

John begins his discourse by talking about the importance of walking in the light. There are two reasons given in verse 7 that tell us why it is important that we walk in the light and live by the truth. What are they?

1. _____

_____

2. _____

_____

What happens if we claim to be without sin (see v. 8)?

_____

_____

_____

_____

On what can we hang our assurance of forgiveness (see v. 9)?

_____

_____

_____

_____

_____

Is there any qualification on the sins God will forgive if we confess our transgressions to Him? Explain your answer.

_____

_____

_____

_____

_____

What does 2 Corinthians 5:17-21 tell us about reconciliation (making peace with God)?

_____

_____

_____

_____

_____

How does what you have learned today affirm this week's memory verse? Write your explanation in the space below. If you need more space, continue writing in your journal.

_____

_____

_____

_____

Merciful Father, thank You that whenever I stumble I can always come to You in contrite confession. Amen.

RECEIVING WHAT GOD HAS GIVEN

Today I give You praise, O gracious Father, for forgiving me of my sins and cleansing me of all unrighteousness. I am truly a new creation in Christ Jesus, and I give You all the glory, honor and praise. Amen.

Many Christians suffer from something called *compound guilt*. The reason is because they have never been able, or perhaps willing, to receive God's forgiveness. It is not that our gracious and merciful God has not forgiven them. When Jesus Christ stretched out His arms on the cross and said, "It is finished" (John 19:30), nothing else was needed. When we confess our sins and trust in Jesus' atonement on our behalf, we are forgiven. The problem lies in our ability to receive what God has so freely given.

What does our memory verse for the week tell us about the connection between forgiveness and hope?

_____

_____

_____

_____

Read Titus 3:3-7. What was our condition before the kindness and love of God our Savior appeared (see vv. 3-4)?

_____

_____

_____

_____

When God our Savior appeared, what did He do (see vv. 5-7)?

_____

_____

_____

_____

_____

According to verses 5 and 7, why did He save us?

_____

_____

_____

_____

How did God save us (see vv. 5-6)?

_____

_____

_____

_____

In a profound mystery that theologians call "substitutionary atonement," Jesus, the righteous One, took on our sins and we received His righteousness. Yet when we refuse to accept the forgiveness Jesus Christ has so freely given us, what are we doing? (Galatians 5:1-6 may help you formulate your answer.)

_____

_____

_____

_____

No matter how destructive your past may have been, there is no reason to carry a burden of guilt and shame. Today, you can hear and believe the good news of the gospel and take it into the depths of your soul. In Christ Jesus, God no longer counts our sins against us! Christ died for us. He rose for us. Christ reigns in power for us. Christ intercedes for us at the right hand of the Father. Our sins have been covered by the blood of the Lamb!

> _Lord, today I acknowledge that nothing, absolutely nothing, could earn what You have freely given me in Jesus Christ. He who knew no sin became sin for me so that I might become the righteousness of God! Amen._

THE BITTER ROOT THAT DEFILES MANY

Merciful God, today I will forgive others because in Jesus Christ You have forgiven me (see Ephesians 4:32). Amen.

At the beginning of this week's study, we saw that there are two inner attitudes that prevent us from having the renewed hope that God longs to give us. One attitude is guilt; the other is bitterness. For the past four days, our lessons have been devoted to the sin-sickness called guilt. Now it is time to tackle the second inner attitude that erodes our hope, what the writer to the Hebrews calls "the bitter root that defiles many." Although bitterness is a complex problem on a human level, the answer to the problem is simple: obedience to the Word of God.

Turn to Hebrews 12 and read verses 14 through 16. In verse 14, we are exhorted to make every effort to live in peace with all men and to be holy. Why is holiness to be our goal (see the last part of v. 14)?

_____

_____

_____

_____

Following the exhortation to be holy, Hebrews 12:15-16 gives us four specific things we are to guard against. What are they?

1. See to it that no one misses the _____ ____ _____.
2. And that no _____ _____ grows up to cause _____
3. See that no one is _____ _____.
4. Or is _____ like Esau.

Now turn to Ephesians 4:31. What does Paul say in this verse?

_____

_____

_____

_____

Once again, note the other things coupled with bitterness in this verse. How would you describe how serious this bitterness problem is?

_____

_____

_____

_____

In Ephesians 4:32, Paul gives us the reason we are not to be bitter about what others have done, or not done, in the past. What does Paul exhort us to be?

Kind and _____ to one another, _____ each other, just as in _____ God forgave you.

How is this truth affirmed in Colossians 3:12-14?

_____

_____

_____

_____

As forgiven sinners, we are to forgive others—not because what they did or didn't do was right, just or fair, but because God in Christ has forgiven us (for all the things that we have done that aren't right, just or fair!). Forgiveness means to forfeit our right to get even. In Romans 12:19-21, Paul tells us the secret to giving up our right to get even with those who have wronged us. What are we to do instead of seeking revenge?

_____

_____

_____

_____

When we insist on carrying around bitterness, rage and anger for what has happened in the past, we are saying that God will not keep His promise;

that He is not the just Judge who will dry every tear and right every wrong. Is this really a statement you want to make to God? Explain your answer.

_____

_____

_____

_____

What bitterness might you be hanging on to that you would like to release to God? (You might want to record your answer in your journal.)

_____

_____

_____

Each time those bitter memories come up again, instead of crying out for revenge, use God's Word to remind yourself that you have chosen to leave vengeance in the hands of the Lord. You have decided to overcome evil with good rather than being overcome by the wiles of the Evil One who seeks your destruction.

O Lord, thank You for Your precious Word! In it You have given me simple solutions to the complex problems that keep me stuck in a downward cycle of defeat and despair. Amen.

Day 6 REFLECTION AND APPLICATION

Gracious God, as a forgiven sinner I will bear with others and forgive those who have sinned against me. I will forgive as You have forgiven me (see Colossians 3:13). Amen.

Sin is not a popular concept in today's society—even among those who call themselves Christians. It is so much easier to disguise our disobedience, calling it a mistake or a human weakness, than to call it what it really is: an offense against a just and holy God. Yet until we reach the point where we are willing to call sin, sin, there is no hope for forgiveness. First John 1:8 and 10 go so far as to say that if we say we have not sinned, then we are not only deceiving ourselves, but we are also calling God a liar! Confession is the only pathway to a restored relationship with God.

For many of us, confession brings up images of groveling and humiliation, being demeaned and shamed because we did not measure up to the unrealistic expectations of others. It can bring up images of admitting to things we did not do because someone else thought they were wrong, or feeling like a failure because we didn't measure up to the world's yardstick. But true confession is none of those things.

Simply put, confession is agreeing with God. Rather than soft-soaping sin and calling God a liar, we tell Him that He was right and we were wrong. Our Father really did know best! Daily confession is an integral part of a right relationship with God. Only when we admit our sins, which separate us from a just and holy God, can we once again be restored to an unbroken fellowship with the source of all goodness and blessing.

What thoughts and images come up for you when you hear the word "confession"?

_____

_____

_____

_____

In what ways is daily confession an integral part of your relationship with God?

_____

_____

_____

_____

Spend some time talking to God about any unwillingness you may have had in the past to be completely honest before Him. Ask Him to send the Holy Spirit, the One who convicts us of our sin and convinces us of Christ's righteousness, to help you understand the truth about confession.

Merciful and loving God, I can leave my tarnished past behind because You no longer count my sins against me. Thank You for a new beginning in Christ Jesus my Lord. Amen.

Day
7

REFLECTION AND APPLICATION

Gracious God, I will sing a new song, because You have done marvelous things (see Psalm 98:1). I will exalt You, my God and King, and praise Your name for ever and ever. Amen.

First Peter 1:3 tells us the reason why we are to give praise to the God and Father of our Lord Jesus Christ. What has God, in His great mercy, done for us?

_____

_____

_____

_____

What is this "new birth" Peter is talking about, and why do you think the apostle calls this hope "living"?

_____

_____

_____

_____

When we live in the hope we have as new creations in Christ Jesus, the whole world becomes our spiritual classroom. So today, rather than doing a head knowledge exercise, we are going to use our hands.

Begin this reflection by finding some pictures that symbolize new birth—a newborn baby, a picture of a baptism, a sprouting seed, a chicken emerging from an egg, a butterfly. Be creative as you look for pictures that, to you, signify the miracle of new life. Collect at least a dozen pictures before you begin this project. You will also need a picture of yourself as you look today.

Once you have collected all the new-life pictures, write the words of this week's memory verse across the top of a piece of paper in bold letters. (You can use heavyweight construction paper for this, but ordinary copy paper works just as well.) After you have written the memory verse, paste the picture of you in the center of the paper and then arrange the other new-life pictures around your picture, making a collage of praise to the God and Father who has given you new birth into a living hope.

Lord, every day I will praise You and extol Your name because You have given me the miracle of new life through Jesus Christ my Lord (see Psalm 145:1-2). I am a precious child of God, a new creation in Christ Jesus, and my sins have been covered by the blood of the Lamb. I praise You, God!

Group Prayer Requests

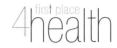

Today's Date: _____

Name	Request

Results

_____

_____

_____

_____

_____

_____

Week Five

hope leads to
action

SCRIPTURE MEMORY VERSE
Be joyful in hope, patient in affliction, faithful in prayer.
ROMANS 12:12

In the past, you might have substituted "wishful thinking" for the genuine hope that leads to positive change. Although you knew that something was wrong, that something needed to change, instead of swinging into action, you might have just hoped things would get better—and then wondered why nothing changed!

As the memory verse for Week Two affirmed, hope deferred makes the heart sick. When wishful thinking is a substitute for hope that leads to action, we are the ones responsible for making our heart sick! Until we begin to bring our attitudes and actions in line with the revealed will of God, hope will continue to elude us. When nothing changes, nothing changes—no matter how wishful our thoughts! Without action, hope is just an illusion that adds to our pain.

Think of a time when you hoped for something that would have made a meaningful contribution to your health journey but perhaps you failed to take action to make your dreams and goals a reality. What was your "hope," and what was the result of hope that was not coupled with action?

_____

_____

_____

_____

WISHING AND PRAYING

Father, help me to never pray lofty prayers and then expect You to do things for me that I am not willing to do for myself. Let me always be humble and look to You as my source of strength. Amen.

While Jesus was here on earth, He taught His disciples a simple prayer that many of us learned in early childhood. It is recited in public worship, in recovery meetings and in public forums. But how many of us follow the words we sometimes mindlessly recite with action that gives credence to our prayer?

Turn in your Bible to Matthew 6:9-13. After carefully reading and praying Jesus' words, begin to compare your everyday actions with the words you have just offered up to God. How have you honored God today as your Father in heaven?

How have you revered His name by caring for yourself in a way that reflects His great love for you?

Have your thoughts and activities been self-indulgent? How have they promoted God's kingdom here on earth?

How have you been content with your "daily bread," the life-giving portion of food that God, in His wisdom, has portioned for you? Or have you eaten more than your share? Describe your thoughts today about your "daily bread."

_____

_____

_____

_____

_____

_____

Have you forgiven others, as God in Christ has forgiven you? Why or why not?

_____

_____

_____

_____

After praying that you not be tempted by the evil one, have you intentionally gone to places where you knew temptation lurked—a restaurant where you habitually overeat, spending time with friends who don't support your health and fitness goals? Have you watched television programs where commercials and indulgent behavior erode your commitment to health and wholeness? Or maybe you've done just the opposite and are aware of how God has protected you from temptation. Either way, describe your state of mind as a result of what you've focused on today.

_____

_____

_____

_____

After completing this exercise, what have you learned about the need for action that is in harmony with the words you offer up to your heavenly Father in prayer?

_____

_____

_____

_____

Lord God Almighty, help me to know when I am powerless and must depend on Your goodness and grace. Help me to not keep myself in defeat but always do the things You have asked me to do. Amen.

Day 2 — SWINGING INTO ACTION

Loving and merciful Father, You call me to affirm Your pleasure when I take action to achieve Your desire for me. Help me to always follow Your will.

Before you begin today's study, spend some time thinking about yesterday's lesson. What did you learn about the connection between hope—even hope that is disguised as prayer—and taking positive action that will bring about the hoped-for change?

_____

_____

_____

_____

How will this knowledge affect the way you approach your First Place 4 Health efforts?

_____

_____

_____

_____

_____

Listed below are the life-changing actions we have examined so far during this study. Complete each of the sentences below by connecting the action verbs on the left with the corresponding phrases on the right.

Accepted — fad diets and instant-results programs are not a God-honoring way to permanent and lasting change.

Obeyed — out to God in our distress, confident that He is our help in time of trouble.

Agreed — to God that we have done things our way and not His.

Cried — God's forgiveness, knowing it is not the gravity of our sin but the greatness of His mercy that matters!

Acknowledged — God's command to rid ourselves of bitterness, leaving vengeance to the One who has promised to right all wrongs.

Matthew 25:14-27 tells us about three servants entrusted with their master's resources. Read those verses and write the words of verse 21 below.

_____

_____

_____

_____

How is the action you have taken thus far in this study part of being a good and faithful servant of our Lord Jesus Christ?

_____

_____

_____

_____

Make the words of Matthew 25:21 your Master's affirmation of your efforts toward achieving the balance, health and wholeness that bring Him glory and honor. Fill in the affirmation with specific words that describe in what you have invested.

_____

_____

_____

_____

Gracious God, thank You for helping me do Your good, pleasing and perfect will when it comes to caring for my body, because You care for me. Amen.

Day 3 BEING JOYFUL, PATIENT AND FAITHFUL

Thank You, Lord, that You give me the strength and the courage to be joyful in hope, patient in affliction, faithful in prayer (see Romans 12:12). Amen.

The memory verse for this week is about taking three simple actions with three specific inner attitudes. Write the three action words and the attitude connected to each one, and then circle the action and attitude that is most difficult for you. What could you do today to practice that inner attitude?

_____

_____

_____

_____

In your own words, explain how joyful hope is different from the deferred hope of Proverbs 13:12.

_____

_____

_____

_____

Turn in your Bible to Isaiah 58:3-5. The people were taking action, but the action was not producing results. What did God tell these people they were doing wrong?

_____

_____

_____

We can often fool ourselves into thinking that we are doing what pleases God. What did God say about this to the prophet Samuel in 1 Samuel 16:7?

_____

_____

_____

_____

How might your inner attitudes be a deterrent to the joyful hope that will produce positive results?

_____

_____

_____

If you were rating your health efforts on a scale of 1 to 10, with 10 being "joyful in hope," and 1 being "just going through the motions," where would you rate yourself?

1   2   3   4   5   6   7   8   9   10

Why did you give yourself that rating, and, more important, what one thing can you do today to become more joyful in hope?

_____

_____

_____

Look back at the memory verse for this week. Explain the connection between joyful hope, patient endurance and faithfulness in prayer. How do these three things work together to bring harmony and balance to your First Place 4 Health efforts?

_____

_____

_____

_____

O Sovereign Lord, You are the one who sees my inner thoughts and attitudes. Today I will not be content to just go through the motions. Instead, I will examine my motives so that what I do and say will find favor in Your eyes.

Day 4 — PERSEVERING WITH PATIENCE

O Lord, I trust in Your unfailing love, confident that You are present in all my circumstances, even those that are not pleasant in the present moment.

Although we tend to think of joy as an emotion and confuse it with happiness, Scripture tells us that joy is an inner attitude that is not dependent on what's happening around us and to us. How do the words "happiness" and "happening" connect, and how does understanding that connection encourage spiritual growth?

_____

_____

_____

_____

How is the joyful hope we have when we consistently take the next step in the right direction different from happiness?

_____

_____

_____

_____

Read James 1:2. What does this Scripture tell us produces pure joy?

_____

_____

_____

_____

How are James's words related to the middle imperative in this week's memory verse?

_____

_____

_____

_____

According to James 1:2-4, how does joyful hope allow us to develop patience?

_____

_____

_____

_____

Now look at James 1:6-7. What does James say about the man or woman who is not patient in affliction?

_____

_____

_____

_____

What happens when we are not patient with the process that leads to our health goals?

_____

_____

_____

_____

First Peter 1:13 admonishes us to prepare our minds for action. Read that verse and then list the two things Peter says we are to do as we prepare our minds:

1. _____

2. _____

List one thing you can do today to prepare your mind for action and one way you can exercise self-control.

_____

_____

_____

_____

_____

Gracious God, on my own I can do no good thing. Thank You for Your Holy Spirit, the One who works in and through me so that I can do Your will. Amen.

Day 5 — RENEWING HOPE WITH PRAYER

Lord God, when I ask for my daily bread and then consume more food than I need to strengthen my body, I know my actions and words are not pleasing to You. Help me today to give my struggles up to You completely. Thank You, Lord. Amen.

Earlier in this study, we looked at the words of the prayer Jesus taught His disciples to pray. Turn to Matthew 6:9-13 and reread these verses. As part of being joyful in hope, patient in affliction and faithful in prayer, we are going to look forward in joyful hope to what we can do to bring our words and actions into harmony when we pray this prayer. As you read the Lord's Prayer, write an attitude or action you will take related to each phrase as part of your program of renewing hope with regard to your health and fitness goals.

Our Father in heaven, hallowed be your name, Your kingdom come, your will be done on earth as it is in heaven. Give us today our daily bread. Forgive us our debts, as we also have forgiven our debtors. And lead us not into temptation but deliver us from the evil one.

Write the words of Psalm 19:14 below.

_____

_____

_____

_____

What consistent action will you take to make your heartfelt prayer a meditation in motion?

_____

_____

_____

_____

Heavenly Father, how grateful I am to be part of the great family of God here on earth. Help me to be a faithful and obedient child and to honor Your name in my actions and attitudes. Amen.

REFLECTION AND APPLICATION

Day 6

Today, O Lord, I will be joyful in hope, patient in affliction, faithful in prayer, because I know that when I do the things that honor You, You guide my steps along the right path. I love You, O Lord, my strength. Amen.

A T-shirt slogan reads, "Lead me not into temptation—I can find it myself." This humorous one-liner raises an interesting question: Do we really mean what we say when we ask not to be led into temptation? If most of us are honest with ourselves, we have to admit that we seldom really want to be delivered from temptation, mainly because temptation promises us way too much fun. Temptation stirs the blood and inflames the imagination. As a matter of fact, if we were revolted by it, it wouldn't be temptation at all.

Occasionally, we are given the grace to see where temptation will take us, and we cry out for deliverance before the fact. But usually temptation doesn't seem all that bad. If temptation brought along chains to bind us, we might be able to resist it on our own. But on the surface, temptation does not appear to be an oppressive force. It is only after we are ensnared that we cry out to God for deliverance from the consequences of our disobedience.

Those of us who are dedicated to health and fitness know just how alluring temptation can appear. Each day we are surrounded by an endless stream of food triggers—on television, in grocery store ads, in magazines and in cookbooks. That is why it is essential to our First Place 4 Health efforts that we pray "and lead us not into temptation" on a daily, and perhaps even a minute-to-minute, basis. After we have prayed, it is important that we do our part by eliminating those temptations that lead us astray. If we invite temptation into our lives, we can't expect to be able to resist.

Part of being delivered from temptation is identifying and eliminating temptations before they have an opportunity to entice us into abandoning our commitment to balanced health. Both prayer and planning are part of our commitment to healthy living. If we do these preparations, God will honor our prayer that we not be led into temptation.

Identify one temptation you can eliminate today and one life-affirming behavior you can put in its place so that your hope will be based on purposeful action, not wishful thinking.

_____

_____

_____

_____

_____

Gracious Lord, thank You for giving me hope that allows me to endure trials patiently. When I pray that Your will is done on earth as it is in heaven, I know that I am vowing to do the things I know You want me to do. Amen.

REFLECTION AND APPLICATION

Father, thank You for speaking to me in a personal way when I meditate on Your Word and talk to You in prayer. You are my God and Father, the One who has given me a living hope in Christ Jesus my Lord. Amen.

The memory verse for this week consists of three short imperatives. Write those imperatives in the space below.

1. _____

2. _____

3. _____

One way to better understand the words of Scripture is to read a verse or phrase out loud, placing emphasis on various words. For reflection today, say your memory verse out loud several times, emphasizing different words each time. Make a note of the words and thoughts that resonate in your soul the most.

_____

_____

_____

_____

Conclude your reflection time by talking to God about the words you have written down. You can be sure that your Father in heaven has a special message for you as you meditate on His words and speak them to Him in prayer.

Today I will praise You, Father, Son and Holy Spirit. Today I will put my hope in God my Savior rather than be downcast, disturbed and in danger of turning back to wishful thinking that does not lead to positive change. Amen.

Group Prayer Requests

4 first place
health

Today's Date: _____

Name	Request

Results

_____
_____
_____
_____
_____

faith ensures hope

Scripture Memory Verse
*Now faith is being sure of what we hope for
and certain of what we do not see.*
Hebrews 11:1

Many people use the word "faith" in the same way they use the word "hope"—as fantasy that their life will get better, even though they fail to take the action steps that will make their hopes and dreams become reality. As we begin our study on the correlation between faith and hope, turn to James 2:14-17. After reading James's command to take action when a brother or sister is in need, paraphrase this idea to apply it to you and your First Place 4 Health program (which is your "need").

When we put faith into action, our faith becomes faith in motion—active faith with practical application. When we turn on a light switch, we have faith that the lights will come on. We do not stop to analyze our actions. We do not need to understand how electrical current works. We do not stand by the light switch and recite a positive affirmation, something like, "I have faith in the electrical wiring in my home; therefore, I will flip the light switch in confidence that I will get light." We simply flip on the switch in faith that we will get light.

Conversely, no matter how great we may claim our faith is in the electrical wiring in our home, unless we take the action (turning on the switch) we will sit in the dark. To paraphrase James's words, "Faith that is not accompanied by action does not provide light for the room!"

Day 1 — FAITH PLEASES GOD

O Lord God, one look at Your creation is all the evidence I need to know that You are the mighty and powerful God You claim to be. Amen.

Our memory verse for the week comes from Hebrews 11, which is about men and women who stepped out in faith in God's leading. Our studies this week will be based on that chapter as we learn what faith in action looks like and then learn to apply those truths to our own efforts toward a healthy lifestyle that is pleasing to God.

In Romans 15:4, the apostle Paul tells us why it is important to study the lives of those who have gone before us. What benefits can you glean from this passage?

_____

_____

_____

_____

_____

How do those benefits contribute to our process of renewing hope?

_____

_____

_____

_____

As you begin this study, notice the words "sure" and "certain" in this week's memory verse. Look up those words in a thesaurus to find synonyms, and write those synonyms in the space below.

_____

_____

_____

_____

_____

Now look up the word "faith." What are synonyms for this word?

_____

_____

_____

_____

Take a few minutes to read all of Hebrews 11, as it will provide a good overview for what we are going to study this week. Now look at Hebrews 11:2. This verse tells us something about the "ancients" and what they were commended for. If God were looking at your faith in action when it comes to practicing the principles of balanced health, would He commend you? Why or why not?

_____

_____

_____

_____

Now look at verse 6. What is it impossible to do without faith?

_____

_____

_____

_____

_____

According to verse 6, what two things do we need to be sure of—to be confident about—in order to have faith that pleases God?

1. _____

2. _____

Are you absolutely certain that God exists and that He will reward you when you earnestly seek Him? Why or why not?

_____

_____

_____

_____

_____

Sovereign Lord, You tell me to ask, seek and knock, confident that You are the giver of all good gifts (see Matthew 7:7). Today I come to You in faith, assured that You will reward my efforts, no matter how feeble I feel they may be. Amen.

Day 2 — FAITH MEANS NOT ASKING WHY

O Lord, I know that You are pleased when I put my faith into action rather than asking questions and doing it my way instead of Yours. Help me to put my faith in action today. Amen.

One characteristic of faith in action is doing exactly what God tells us to do, even when we don't fully understand the reason why. Let's resume our study of Hebrews 11 by turning to verse 7. What did Noah do?

_____

_____

_____

_____

To learn more about Noah's faith, look at Genesis 6:9-22. What did God tell Noah to do, and why (see vv. 14-17)?

_____

_____

_____

_____

_____

In giving Noah instruction, God was very specific about some things and vague about others. What does this tell you about the way God gives us instruction, even today?

_____

_____

_____

_____

_____

Genesis 6:22 shows us an important aspect of faith in action. What does this verse tell us about Noah's faith?

_____

_____

_____

_____

_____

In Genesis 7:4, God told Noah when the rain would begin and how long it would last. When it began to rain, what did Noah do (see v. 13)?

_____

_____

_____

_____

_____

In some ways, your First Place 4 Health story parallels Noah's faith experience. What specific details has God given you about what you are to include in your efforts to take better care of yourself? What part of this journey is still vague to you?

_____

_____

_____

_____

_____

If Noah were sitting in the room with you today, what would you ask him about his faith in action?

_____

_____

_____

_____

_____

Faithful Father, thank You for men and women of faith, and for including each of their stories in the Bible. Their faith stories teach me how to endure so that through the encouragement of the Scriptures I might have hope (see Romans 15:4). Amen.

Day 3 — FAITH ANTICIPATES A FUTURE OF HOPE

O Lord, so often I don't see the path in front of me. Thank You that Your Word gives me eyes of faith that allow me to do Your will so that I can achieve Your purpose for me. Amen.

There's another important aspect of faith in action, a living faith that is not based on false hopes and pipe dreams. Turn to Hebrews 11:22 and read the short account from the life of Joseph. In order to fully comprehend the depth of Joseph's faith, we must turn back to Genesis 50:24-25.

What did Joseph say to his brothers in these verses, and what did he make the sons of Israel swear on an oath to do?

_____

_____

_____

_____

_____

Now turn to Genesis 15:12-14. What do you learn from these verses that can help you to better understand Joseph's faith-filled instructions to his brothers?

_____

_____

_____

_____

How long did God say the Israelites would be enslaved and mistreated (see v. 13)? What does this tell you about the patience in affliction spoken of in our memory verse from Week Five?

_____

_____

_____

_____

Read 2 Peter 1:3-4. What adjectives does the apostle Peter use to describe God's promises?

_____

_____

_____

_____

How are God's promises part of the good gifts He gives us so that we can live a life pleasing to Him (see v. 3)?

_____

_____

_____

_____

What else do these great and precious promises allow us to do (see v. 4)?

_____

_____

_____

_____

When we consider what God said to Abraham and then what Joseph believed as a result of that promise, what lesson can we learn about the importance of reading, knowing and memorizing God's Word?

_____

_____

_____

_____

Write one Scripture verse from memory in the space below. Explain how that verse can be an integral part of your faith in action as you journey toward the health and wholeness that is pleasing to God.

_____

_____

_____

_____

_____

Gracious Father, I am humbled when I read the stories of the men and women of faith. Help me trust in You so that I, too, can become one of the great cloud of witnesses cheering for others just beginning the race. Amen.

FAITH MEANS NOT LOOKING BACK

Lord, help me to let go of any faulty beliefs so that I can hear the truth of Your Word and do everything just as You tell me to do it. Amen.

In the midst of the stories of faith in Hebrews 11, there is one little verse that we often overlook. Read verse 15 and describe what this verse says about faith in action.

_____

_____

_____

Jesus also talked about this important faith-in-action principle to His followers. Read Luke 9:62 to learn what Jesus said about not looking back, and then explain this in your own words.

_____

_____

_____

Paul, in Philippians 3:12-14, affirms this same truth by using the analogy of a runner. What does Paul tell us in those verses?

_____

_____

_____

When Paul brought the gospel of Jesus Christ to the people of Ephesus, some of the people took bold action so that they would not return to their old beliefs. Read Acts 19:19. What happened?

_____

_____

_____

From what you have learned in today's lesson, why is letting go of faulty thinking such an important principle?

_____

_____

_____

_____

What old beliefs do you need to let go of so that you can take the faith-in-action steps that will result in pursuing balanced nutrition and sensible exercise?

_____

_____

_____

_____

Sovereign Lord, I know that the plans You have for me are good. Help me to realize those perfect plans by stepping out in faith, believing in Your Word and trusting that Your great and precious promises are yes and amen in Jesus Christ. Amen.

Day 5 — FAITH OVERCOMES THE PAST

Gracious God, I have seen the importance of stepping out in faith and doing exactly what You ask me to do. Help me leave my past behind so that I can realize the wonderful things You have in store for me. Amen.

At first glance, there is one name that seems out of place in the line-up of the giants of the faith: Rahab. Turn to Hebrews 11:31 and write down what you learn about Rahab from this brief snippet about her life.

_____

_____

_____

_____

To learn more about Rahab, turn to Joshua 2 and read of her faith in action despite her checkered past. Who did this woman of faith defy in order to protect the spies (see v. 3)? Rather than turning in the spies, what did Rahab do (see vv. 4-7)?

_____

_____

_____

_____

Joshua 2:8-13 tells us why Rahab was courageous enough to put her faith into action. What do these verses tell you about her view of God, even though she was not part of the visible family of God?

_____

_____

_____

_____

What does Rahab's faith teach us about making assumptions that are connected to a person's profession, ethnicity, culture, language or race (see 1 Samuel 16:7)?

_____

_____

_____

_____

Because of her faith in action, Rahab occupies a special place in salvation history. Turn to Matthew 1:5. In what family lineage do you see her name listed? Why is this significant?

_____

_____

_____

_____

No matter what your family background, personal history or heritage might be, what plans might God have for you that you will only realize by stepping out in faith and taking action that gives credence to your profession of faith?

_____

_____

_____

_____

_____

Spend some time today thanking God for the wonderful plans He has for you—plans that aren't dependent on your present circumstances or on your past. Ask God to tell you what you must do in order to make those plans come to fruition, and as you meditate on His Word, listen for His answer!

O Lord God Almighty, thank You that Your mercy and grace are stronger than anything in my past. I turn to You in faith and put my hope and trust in You today, tomorrow and for all of my tomorrows, until I am taken to heaven to live with You throughout eternity. Amen.

Day 6

REFLECTION AND APPLICATION

Lord God, help me be a fruitful and faithful servant who does everything just as You tell me to do it! Amen.

During our lessons this week, we have examined the lives of four men and women of faith who are listed in Hebrews 11. Yet there are many wonderful faith-in-action stories in this chapter that our study did not include. Today is your opportunity to learn more about another man or woman of faith listed among the faithful in Hebrews 11.

Go back and reread that chapter, making note of the person whose story the Holy Spirit brings to your awareness in a special way. Perhaps it is just a short word or phrase that attracts you to this person's faith story. Next, using a Bible concordance, find out what you can discover about the man or woman whose story the Spirit has prompted you to learn more about. Then go to the chapter(s) in which his or her story appears to read about that person's life and faith.

Be prepared to present this giant of the faith to your First Place 4 Health group during your next meeting. In addition to just the facts about this person, be ready to tell your group what this person's story taught you that will help you put your faith in action too.

> *To You, O Lord, I lift up my soul; in You I trust, O my God. Guide me in*
> *Your truth and teach me, for You are God my Savior, and my hope is in*
> *You all day long (see Psalm 25:1-2,5).*

REFLECTION AND APPLICATION

Day 7

> *Sovereign Lord, I pray today that You will never let me substitute wishful*
> *thinking for genuine faith that results in action—action that does what You*
> *tell me to do, even when I don't understand why and can't see*
> *where my steps will lead me. Thank You, Lord. Amen.*

"Euphoric recall" is a term used to describe a selective memory process that allows recovering addicts to recall how good they felt when they were using their drug of choice—but somehow forget how foolishly they behaved and the dire consequences of their behavior. Because of euphoric recall, memories of "how it was" are always filtered through distorted perceptions.

Remembering how good the high felt in the absence of recalling the painful consequences can keep addicts from fully realizing the unmanageability of their disease and the depth of their addiction. As a result, euphoric recall limits these addicts' ability to truly admit their powerlessness and their total dependence on God to deliver them from their addiction.

However, euphoric recall isn't a present-day phenomenon limited just to recovering addicts! Euphoric recall was the downfall of many individuals in the Bible who thought about where they would come from rather than looking forward to where they were going with eyes of faith. Throughout the book of Exodus, we see that the children of Israel, when faced with a period of testing in the desert, began to suffer from euphoric recall. They remembered the good, "free" food they had in Egypt, when in reality they had paid a very high price for that food: bondage and slavery. They remembered the meat, cucumbers, melons, leeks, onions and garlic, but not the cruel taskmasters who oppressed and mistreated them. They remembered the pleasure but forgot all about the pain.

Many of us who are striving to achieve balance, health and wholeness also fall into the euphoric recall trap. We remember the delicacies we ate before healthy living became a priority. We recall how good the food that eroded our wellbeing tasted, but we neglect to remember the price tag attached to the pleasure. We talk about how we used to be able to do things that do not fit into our new self-disciplined lifestyle, and we forget about the high price we paid for the privilege of indulging in self-destructive behavior. How quickly we remember the pleasure—how quickly we forget the pain our out-of-control behavior caused.

Today, rather than looking back at what we had when we were in bondage to our cravings, let's step forward in faith! Let's remember the life we now enjoy because we are putting God first in all things and reaping His abundant blessings.

In what ways, if any, is euphoric recall undermining your commitment to live the First Place 4 Health lifestyle?

_____

_____

_____

_____

_____

What have you learned from the men and women of faith in this week's Bible study that will help you to leave the past in the past so that you can press on to the prize that only those who take action steps in faith will enjoy?

_____

_____

_____

_____

_____

_____

Thank God for showing you the truth about your destructive past and giving you examples from His Word on how you can step forward in faith.

> *Lord, Your Word is a lamp to my feet and a light to my path (see Psalm 119:105). Help me step out in faith, not considering the cost and not looking back, but putting my hand to the plow because I have heard Jesus say, "Follow Me." Amen.*

Group Prayer Requests

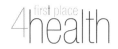

Today's Date: ....

Name	Request

Results

....

....

....

....

....

....

knowledge increases hope

SCRIPTURE MEMORY VERSE
Find rest, O my soul, in God alone; my hope comes from him.
PSALM 62:5

We have covered a lot of ground in the past few weeks, and by now you are realizing that hope is more than wishful thinking. Hope is purposeful action that requires taking the next right step in the right direction, confident that the God of hope is the One directing your steps and setting your course.

Before we continue with our study, take a time-out to put a word we find sprinkled throughout the psalms into practice. Turn in your Bible to Psalm 62, the psalm from which this week's memory verse is taken. To the right of the last word in verse 4 you will see a word set apart from the rest of the text. (It also appears after verse 8.) That word, "Selah," in our twenty-first-century vernacular, means "Stop and think about it." This is exactly what we are going to do before we move into this week's study.

As you contemplate what you have learned about hope thus far, write the three words or phrases that immediately come to your mind when you complete the sentence "Hope is . . ."

1. _____
2. _____
3. _____

What have you learned about the relationship between hope and action?

_____

_____

_____

_____

What is the difference between deferred hope and joyful hope? Compare these two very different kinds of hope with the other.

_____

_____

_____

_____

Day 1

STOP AND THINK ABOUT IT

Gentle and loving Lord, thank You for inviting me to take Your yoke upon me and learn from You. I look forward in joyful hope to the lessons You would have me learn. Amen.

As we take a few moments to stop and think about what we have learned thus far, let us add some words Jesus spoke to those who were weary and burdened, those who had been in a position of deferred hope for way too long and for whom the weight of the oppression was almost more than they could bear. Turn to Matthew 11 and read verses 25 through 30. As you read, think about what Jesus is saying. You might want to reread the passage, letting the words sink into the depths of your weary soul.

From whom has the knowledge of the kingdom of God been hidden (see Matthew 11:25)?

_____

_____

_____

_____

To whom has the knowledge of the Kingdom been revealed, and whose good pleasure was it to do things this way (see vv. 25-26)?

_____

_____

_____

_____

What knowledge has the Father committed to Jesus (the living Word of God) that the world does not possess, and with whom is He willing to share it (see v. 27)?

_____

_____

_____

_____

What does Jesus invite those who are weary and burdened to do (see v. 28)? (Note that Jesus is talking about weariness of soul, a fatigue that is not relieved by a good night's rest.)

_____

_____

_____

_____

In opposition to the heavy burden of the world, what does Jesus offer (see v. 30)?

_____

_____

_____

_____

Spend the rest of your study time today thanking Jesus for inviting you to share His gentle yoke and to learn from Him. As you learn more about God, you will discover that your hope is being renewed as part of this learning process—and that is always reason for thanks and praise!

> *I praise You, Father, Lord of heaven and earth, because You have chosen to reveal the truth about the kingdom of God to those who are willing to come to You as dependent children. Amen.*

Day 2 ADD TO YOUR FAITH

O Lord God, it is my earnest desire to grow in the grace and knowledge of my Lord and Savior Jesus Christ so that I can give Him glory both now and forever (see 2 Peter 3:17-18). Amen.

The apostle Peter was one of the Twelve who accompanied Jesus as He ministered and taught those who were weary, heavy laden and in need of His healing touch. Like many of us, Peter had lots of enthusiasm and gusto, but he was often slow to learn the important lessons Jesus wanted to teach him.

Perhaps that is why knowledge was so important to Peter as he ministered to the flock the Lord had entrusted to the apostle's care. Today we are going to look at another essential element of renewed hope: *knowledge*—but not just any type of knowledge, and certainly not the knowledge prized by the wise and learned of the world.

Turn to 2 Peter 1:3. What is the specific knowledge that gives us everything we need for life and godliness?

Knowledge of _____ who _____ us by his own _____ and goodness.

In 2 Peter 1:5-7, Peter lists eight qualities we are to possess in increasing measure. List them in the order you find them in Peter's writing.

1. _____
2. _____
3. _____
4. _____
5. _____
6. _____
7. _____
8. _____

What does the phrase "increasing measure" tell you about these qualities?

_____
_____
_____
_____

Why do you think Peter lists knowledge before self-control and self-control before perseverance?

_____
_____
_____
_____

Second Peter 1:8 tells us that if we possess these qualities in increasing measure, they will keep us from being ineffective and unproductive. How might being ineffective and unproductive be part of deferred hope?

_____
_____
_____
_____

In 2 Peter 1:9, Peter goes on to say that anyone who doesn't possess these qualities in increasing measure "is _____ and _____, and has _____ that he has been _____ from his

_____ _____." In what way do Peter's words reinforce how accepting God's forgiveness is part of renewing our hope?

_____

_____

_____

Second Peter ends with Peter's words to his dear friends. As a follower of the Lord Jesus Christ, you are one of the dear friends to whom Peter is speaking. Read his words, found in 2 Peter 3:17-18, as a personal message from one who learned his lessons the hard way, much like most of us do!

> *Jesus, You came to teach me about the Father. Today I will meditate on Your Word and apply the lessons You show me to my life. Amen.*

Day 3

LEARN PRACTICAL KNOWLEDGE

O Lord, You are kind and You are loving. You do not want anyone to perish. Thank You for sending Jesus to teach me the truth about Your tender mercy and love. Amen.

When Jesus was here on earth, He taught His disciples valuable lessons about the kingdom of God, His Father in heaven and His mission to save God's people from their sins. Often Jesus taught these vital lessons by using simple stories called parables. The word "parable" means "to lay alongside in order to compare," and that is exactly what Jesus did in these earthly stories that taught spiritual truth. We can add to our knowledge of God's storehouse by reading these stories and allowing Jesus, the Master Teacher, to be our teacher too.

One of Jesus' parables that, when properly understood, can be part of our journey toward renewed hope is found in Luke 13:6-9. Turn to those verses and read them now. As with all Jesus' parables, this story was told to answer a specific question or clarify a statement Jesus had just made.

What is the statement in Luke 13:5 that prompted this parable about repentance?

_____

_____

_____

_____

_____

What does the parable in Luke 13:6-9 tell us about the fig tree?

_____

_____

_____

_____

_____

Why did the vineyard owner plant the fig tree in his garden? (What is the purpose for which the fig tree was created?)

_____

_____

_____

Likewise, why did the heavenly Vineyard Owner plant you where you are in life, and how does this relate to your First Place 4 Health group?

_____

_____

_____

_____

The fact that the fig tree was purposely planted in a fertile vineyard is important to our comprehension of the lesson being taught. To better understand, turn to Isaiah 5:1-7. After reading the passage, what new knowledge do you have that increases your understanding of the parable Jesus taught about the fig tree?

_____

_____

_____

_____

Has God given you every advantage to be fruitful where you are in your life and in your First Place 4 Health program? Explain your answer.

_____

_____

_____

Many of God's "planted" people were not producing the "fruit of repentance"—they were barren when it came to doing the things that pleased God. But the gardener pleaded with the vineyard owner for one more year—a year of favor to try to stimulate the tree to produce fruit pleasing to God. Who was the One sent to proclaim the year of the Lord's favor, the One who would fertilize and dig around the plant before it was chopped down (see Luke 4:14-21)?

_____

_____

_____

_____

What new knowledge have you gleaned about the Lord Jesus Christ from our study of this parable, and how can this knowledge be part of your renewed hope?

_____

_____

_____

_____

As we conclude our study for today, turn to 2 Peter 3:8-9. After reading Peter's words, spend some time thanking God that you are living in the year of the Lord's favor and that through the power of the Holy Spirit, God is transforming you into a faithful, fruitful servant.

Gracious God, I confess that You have planted me in a fertile vineyard and given me every opportunity to bear fruit for You. Help me seek You and do what You created me to do. Amen.

GROW IN KNOWLEDGE Day 4

Gracious Lord, You are the just judge, the One who is always willing to hear our case and who promises to administer justice for Your people. Thank You for Your promises and Your Word. Amen.

Today we are going to look at another of Jesus' teaching parables, a story that is called a "how much more" parable. The parable we examined yesterday taught us truths about God by using an example that the common folk of Jesus' day would have readily understood. The vineyard owner represented God, the gardener represented Jesus and the fig tree was God's barren, fruitless people. Today's "how much more" parable is different in that it shows us a man who neither fears God nor cares about men, yet still administers justice. Jesus uses this judge as a way of showing us how much more our Father in heaven will bring justice to those who cry out to Him day and night.

Today's parable is found in Luke 18:1-9. Read that story now, making careful note of both characters. Who are the two people in this parable?

What does the parable tell us about the judge?

_____

_____

_____

_____

What does it tell us about the widow?

_____

_____

_____

_____

Although some modern translations use the word "persistent" to describe the woman who is being deprived of justice, older translations use the word "importunate." Look up the word "importunate" in a dictionary and write the meanings given for the word in the space provided.

_____

_____

_____

_____

The unjust judge was neither a God-fearer nor a people-pleaser. Who was the only one this fellow cared about (see v. 5)?

_____

_____

_____

_____

What prompted him to administer justice for the widow?

_____

_____

_____

_____

Although this parable has been misinterpreted to mean we must badger God with our prayers, much like a demanding child wears down a parent with persistent requests, when we interpret this parable in light of the whole counsel of God, we know that nothing we could ever say or do would cause God to violate His character and nature. If this parable is not telling us to badger God, what is it teaching us?

_____

_____

_____

_____

_____

What new thing have you learned from today's study about your responsibility before God as it relates to taking proper care of yourself? How does that honor God?

_____

_____

_____

_____

The parable of the persistent widow ends with a piercing question: "When the Son of Man comes, will he find faith on the earth?" (Luke 18:8). How is persistent prayer an active expression of our faith?

_____

_____

_____

_____

Almighty God, I will be persistent in prayer, crying out to You day and night, confident that You are the giver of all good gifts who hears my cries and is concerned for my wellbeing. Amen.

LEARN THROUGH RHYTHM

O Lord, You have searched me and You know me. How thankful I am that even though You know everything about me, You still love me! Amen.

Although theologians teach us about God with words that are often difficult to understand, there is another way we can learn about the character and nature of God: from the rhythm and cadence of the psalms. Read Psalm 139, making a note of the things it reveals to you about God. Use the space provided to record your findings.

_____

_____

_____

_____

_____

Which verses give you hope of God's ongoing protection? Why?

_____

_____

_____

Which verses give you hope in God's perpetual provision? Why?

_____

_____

_____

_____

Which verses give you hope of God's continual presence, no matter where you are or what you are doing? Why?

_____

_____

_____

Which verses give you hope because God will always be faithful? Why?

_____

_____

_____

_____

Which verses give you hope because they show that you are precious and dearly loved by God? Which give you hope because they show how God will continue to guide you in right paths? Why?

_____

_____

_____

_____

How can what you learned today become part of the hope you have as you care for your wonderfully made body that God created and sustains? Use your journal to record your thoughts.

Gracious God, You created me, You sustain me, You redeemed me. I belong to You. Today I will care for my body because I was purchased at a price— the price of Jesus' precious blood. Amen.

REFLECTION AND APPLICATION   Day 6

Lord, thank You that all Your ways are loving and faithful for those who keep the demands of Your covenant (see Psalm 25:10). Amen.

Today we are going from psalm to psalm on a knowledge-seeking treasure hunt. Listed below are 10 attributes of God. You will look for verses in the psalms that represent each of these 10 attributes.

Begin the treasure hunt by listing the 10 attributes on separate pieces of paper or 3x5-inch cards. Next, look for verses in the book of Psalms that match that attribute. For example, if one of the attributes were "compassion," you might select Psalm 103:13 as the verse that matches that attribute. (Psalm 103:13 tells us, "As a father has compassion on his children, so the Lord has compassion on those who fear him.") When you find a verse that matches the attribute you are searching for, write it on the paper or card containing that attribute.

You can only get one attribute from each psalm you visit, and you can use a psalm verse only one time. Be sure not to use verses from Psalm 139, as we learned lessons from that psalm yesterday. Be prepared to share your knowledge-seeking treasure hunt answers with your First Place 4 Health group the next time you meet.

Attribute	Verse	Attribute	Verse
Justice		Might and power	
Tender mercy		Gentleness	
Unconditional love		Vengeance	
Righteousness		Faithfulness	
Generosity		Sovereignty	

As a bonus question, identify one more attribute of God not on the printed list and find a verse that supports it.

O Lord my God, I called to You for help and You healed me (see Psalm 30:2). I love You, O Lord, my strength. You are my rock, my fortress and my deliverer, my rock in whom I take refuge (see Psalm 18:1-2). Amen.

REFLECTION AND APPLICATION

O Lord, our Lord, how majestic is Your name in all the earth (see Psalm 8:1)! The heavens declare Your glory, O God; the skies proclaim the work of Your hands (see Psalm 19:1). Amen.

We've already discussed that parables are simple stories that use things common folks can easily understand as a way of teaching spiritual truth. Drawing from Jesus' example of using nature as our teacher, today we are going to leave our books and papers behind and go for a nature-walk treasure hunt. Wear comfortable clothing and take a tote bag to collect your treasures. Unlike our treasure hunt yesterday, there will not be a list of things you must find. You will be the one determining what treasures to put in your bag.

As you walk in God's beautiful creation, look for items in nature that teach you something about God, especially as it applies to the God of hope who is continually creating and re-creating His world and the people who occupy it. As you pick up each item and put it into your tote bag, say, "This _____ increases my knowledge about God because _____." Try to find at least seven items, and be prepared to share your findings with your First Place 4 Health group.

May the words of my mouth and the meditation of my heart be pleasing in Your sight, O Lord, my Rock and my Redeemer (see Psalm 19:14). Amen.

Group Prayer Requests

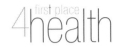

Today's Date: _____

Name	Request

Results

_____

_____

_____

_____

_____

_____

obedience builds hope

Our memory verse for this week asks an important question that also incorporates the idea of *just as the Lord commands*. Read the memory verse as a question to you, and then give the Lord your prayerful answer, especially as doing what He says applies to faithfully following your goal toward health and balance through participation in First Place 4 Health.

_____
_____
_____
_____
_____
_____

SIMPLE INSTRUCTIONS Day 1

Lord, Your words are not trivial; they are my life. I thank You for giving me instruction that I can easily understand and obey (see Deuteronomy 32:47).

This week, we will learn about the things that stand between us and doing what we know to be the next right thing—the step to take or the attitude to cultivate—by looking at the life of a man called Naaman.

Before we begin that study, look up the word "simple" in a dictionary. Write the definition below.

_____

_____

_____

_____

Those are hardly the words you would expect to be used to describe the awesome, powerful Word of God! Yet when all is said and done, that is exactly what God's Word consists of: simple instruction for a simple people, called to live simply so that they can love and serve their Lord with all their heart, soul, mind and strength. How do the words of Moses in Deuteronomy 30:11-14 affirm that God's instructions to us are simple?

_____

_____

_____

_____

We often look for complicated solutions to the problems that plague us rather than obeying God's simple instructions. What does Moses tell us about God's Word in Deuteronomy 32:47?

_____

_____

_____

_____

To conclude today's study, read the story of Naaman found in 2 Kings 5:1-14. (We will discuss what this passage has to teach us in tomorrow's study, so for today just read the story.) Note that Aram is modern-day Syria, so you might want to look up Syria on a map to see it in relation to Israel. Also note that the Israelites and the Syrians were enemies and Naaman was not a God-fearing Jew. What does that tell you about God's love, mercy and grace?

_____

_____

_____

_____

Gracious God, today I will dare to listen as You ask me the question "Why do you call me 'Lord, Lord' and do not do what I say?" (see Luke 6:46). Amen.

POWER OF WITNESS TO OTHERS Day 2

O Lord, my hope often comes through the simple words of others who tell me of the wonderful things You have done for them. Help me to be a witness to Your glory and grace as I speak with others. Amen.

At the conclusion of yesterday's lesson, you read the story of Naaman in 2 Kings 5:1-14. Review his story as we begin today's lesson, and then keep your Bible open to that passage. What do we learn about Naaman in verse 1? List all the facts about him.

_____

_____

_____

_____

There is one thing that seems out of place in this list of stellar accomplishments. Circle that one thing. We glean additional information about Naaman in verse 2: He had a wife, and Israelite slaves were used in his household. How were these slaves acquired?

_____

_____

_____

_____

We learn another piece of information about this general in verse 5. What does the verse tell us?

_____

_____

_____

_____

_____

What else do we learn about Naaman in verse 9?

_____

_____

_____

_____

So, we have a wealthy man who was rich enough to take lavish gifts with him as he traveled to Israel. This powerful man had an entourage of chariots and horses—and there were servants who traveled with him as he journeyed to see the prophet in Samaria. But Naaman's hope of healing didn't come from his wealth or his possessions or his position. From where did his hope come (see 2 Kings 5:2-3)?

_____

_____

_____

_____

What does this tell you about the power of our simple witness to others about the might and power of God?

_____

_____

_____

_____

What simple words of encouragement might God be prompting you to say to someone who may be in need of God's healing touch?

_____

_____

_____

_____

End today's study by writing that person a note of encouragement!

Praise the Lord, O my soul; all my inmost being, praise His holy name. Praise the Lord, O my soul, and forget not all His benefits. He forgives all my sins and heals all my diseases (see Psalm 103:1-3)! Amen.

EXPECTATIONS

Day 3

O Lord God, I know that I must look to You to lose excess weight and follow Your simple instructions. Help me to do that today. Amen.

As we resume our study of Naaman today, review his story in 2 Kings 5:1-14, and, as before, keep your Bible open to this passage. In response to the slave girl's words in verse 3, Naaman gathered expensive gifts to take to the prophet in Samaria. Why do you think Naaman thought it necessary to shower with gifts the man he hoped would heal him?

_____

_____

_____

_____

What does the apostle Paul tell us about God's grace in Ephesians 2:2-10?

_____

_____

_____

_____

Do you think what a person has in terms of material wealth, position or personal power puts him or her in a better position before God than those who do not have these things? Explain your answer.

_____

_____

_____

_____

_____

As Naaman traveled to Samaria, he had an expectation of what would happen when he laid his gifts at the prophet's feet. Read 2 Kings 5:11 and rewrite that sentence in your own words. What happened instead (see v. 10)?

_____

_____

_____

_____

_____

How might part of our deferred hope be the result of expecting a miracle rather than accepting God's simple instructions and following the process He has outlined for our healing?

_____

_____

_____

_____

How might First Place 4 Health be part of that healing process?

_____

_____

_____

_____

When things did not go according to Naaman's expectations, what did he do (see v. 11)?

_____

_____

_____

_____

What were Elisha's instructions? What was Naaman's excuse for not obeying those words (see vv. 10-12)?

_____

_____

_____

_____

What did the servants say to Naaman that brought him back to his senses (see v. 13)?

_____

_____

_____

_____

Think for a moment about the elaborate things you might have done in the name of losing weight—things that might have been complicated, expensive and time-consuming, not to mention counterproductive. What wisdom can you glean from the simple words of Naaman's servants?

_____

_____

_____

_____

What happened when Naaman followed Elisha's instructions just as they were given (see v. 14)?

_____

_____

_____

_____

What can you learn from Naaman's story about the value and importance of obedience?

_____

_____

_____

_____

Sovereign Lord, forgive me for coming to You with any preconceived expectations rather than acknowledging You as the giver of all good gifts, the One who knows what I need even before I ask. Amen.

Day
4

OBSTACLES TO RENEWED HOPE

Gracious God, You have redeemed me because of Your unfailing love, not because of anything I have done to earn Your grace. Thank You, Lord. Amen.

As we have examined an event from the life of Naaman during this week's studies, we have seen how God's simple instructions brought about healing. Naaman's leprous skin was restored because he did exactly what Elisha, the man of God, told him to do. Yet there was another miracle that occurred in this story. Naaman also had some inner attitudes that were cleansed.

Today we are going to look at the six attitudes that almost kept Naaman from receiving the gift of new life. These six attitudes are listed below, adapted to fit our First Place 4 Health situation. After each attitude, note the Scripture reference in 2 Kings 5:1-14 that talks about Naaman's faulty attitude or the things in Naaman's life that contributed to that attitude. Next, talk to God about how the same obstacles might be keeping you from fully doing the Lord's will and reaping the benefit of obedience.

Attitude	Verse	Attitude	Verse
Personal power because of your position		Pride that keeps you from accepting simple solutions	
Accompishments and performance at work, home and at church		Wanting to do what is pleasurable rather than what is necessary	
Material possessions and personal wealth		Petulance that immediately decides God is wrong and you are right	

Summarize what you have learned about restoration from looking at the obstacles that almost kept Naaman from receiving God's help.

_____

_____

_____

_____

How can doing this exercise give you new hope that our gracious God will heal you—body, soul, mind and spirit—as you are obedient to His Word?

_____

_____

_____

_____

Forgive me, Sovereign Lord, for any times that I have become angry with You because You did not agree with my plans, rather than being willing to submit myself completely to Your perfect plan for my life. Amen.

POWERLESSNESS

Gracious and loving Lord, Your grace is sufficient for me, no matter what problem I might face. I will trust in You and not be afraid. Amen.

As we have seen in this week's study, Naaman was a valiant soldier who was highly regarded by those around him. He was a commander of the army of the king of Aram and was considered a great man in his master's sight. He was wealthy and possessed many horses, chariots, servants and other symbols of wealth. Yet he also had a problem that all his wealth and power could not overcome: Naaman had leprosy.

Like it or not, our problem—that thing we are powerless to overcome in our own strength and power—is often the thing that brings us to the point of being willing to listen to God's simple instructions. What are you currently powerless to change without God's grace? (Most of us have many things that we are powerless to control, so make your answer relevant to First Place 4 Health issues.)

_____

_____

_____

_____

The apostle Paul also had an ailment over which he was powerless. Read 2 Corinthians 12:7-10. What was this ailment (see v. 7)?

_____

_____

_____

_____

Whether the "thorn in the flesh" that Paul describes in 2 Corinthians 12:7-10 was a physical condition or spiritual persecution, he was able to bring healing to others, even when he could not help himself. What simple instructions did God, in His grace, give to Paul (see v. 8)?

_____

_____

_____

What inner attitude did Naaman's leprosy allow him to overcome that is akin to the problem of boasting?

_____

_____

Unlike Naaman, Paul did not receive physical healing. What was the solution God gave Paul instead of healing (see v. 9)?

_____

_____

_____

When Naaman first heard God's simple instructions, he got angry and left. How did Paul do it differently (see vv. 9-10)?

_____

_____

_____

How might God be using any powerlessness you might feel over compulsive eating or not taking proper care of yourself as a means of grace in your life?

_____

_____

_____

_____

What part of this week's study has given you renewed hope and new willingness to do everything just as the Lord commands, especially when it comes to doing those things that will allow you to achieve the balance and health possible through participation in First Place 4 Health?

_____

_____

_____

_____

Sovereign Lord, thank You for problems that bring me to the point of accepting Your will and Your Word. When I am powerless, You are all-powerful!

Day 6 REFLECTION AND APPLICATION

Lord, help me to never rely on my own abilities and accomplishments, but to look to Your mercy, grace and love. When I try to purchase Your love, I cheapen Your grace. Amen.

Although your personal history and current circumstance are uniquely your own, there is one thing all human beings have in common: The last thing we surrender to God is an admission of our helplessness to save ourselves. We will give up our vices, our ambitions, our money, our name, our comfort, willing to surrender them all to God. But the most difficult sacrifice—the last stronghold—that we give up is our confidence that there is something we can do that will earn us a right relationship with God.

God is not pleased when we attempt to substitute "righteousness by achievement through performance" for "salvation by grace through faith." He will not allow us to change the terms He has set for an acceptable, pleasing relationship with Him, which can only be had by faith in the atonement made possible through Jesus Christ, our Lord. Yes, we can and should do things that we know are pleasing to God once we are in a right relationship with Him. But we cannot get into a right relationship, no matter how pleasing our behavior, by any means other than faith in Jesus Christ and His substitutionary death that paid the penalty for our sins. If we could earn it, salvation would not be a gift!

Paul wrote, "For it is by grace you have been saved, through faith—and this not from yourselves, it is the gift of God—not by works, so that no one can boast" (Ephesians 2:8-9). God will not share His glory. He will not allow us to claim any credit for our salvation. Grace is a free gift or it isn't grace at all. The moment we try to earn it or pay for it, it ceases to be grace.

Working toward a healthy and balanced life through the First Place 4 Health program is pleasing to God, yet we must be careful to never confuse any spiritual practice with God's grace. We work *from* our salvation, not *for* our salvation. Even as we work to achieve health and balance, we must realize that salvation is a gift.

Have you accepted the gift of salvation that God longs to freely give you? Explain your answer.

_____

_____

_____

_____

Is your participation in the First Place 4 Health program part of your striving to earn salvation, or is it motivated by a sincere desire to please the One who has saved you by grace, and by grace alone? Explain your answer.

_____

_____

_____

_____

These are serious questions that deserve careful consideration. Use today as a day to ponder. As thoughts come, record them in your journal.

Gracious God, You tell me that Your grace is sufficient for me. Thank You for this comfort and consolation when I am in need of Your healing touch. Amen.

REFLECTION AND APPLICATION

Today I will sing for joy to You, O God of Jacob! I will sing Your praise for You have been good to me (see Psalm 81:1). Amen.

Belgian physicist and Nobel Prize winner Ilya Prigogine developed a fascinating theory about a "bigger monkey wrench" that restores order to disordered systems—and disordered lives. Using atomic technology, Prigogine showed that the stimulus for creating order out of disorder is exactly the opposite of what we might imagine it would be.

While we tend to avoid things that cause too much disturbance, Prigogine discovered that throwing a bigger monkey wrench into the works actually stimulates the creation of new structures at an atomic level and produces a profound paradigm shift on a personal level. Prigogine's theory of dissipative structures states that small stressors in a system flatten out, swamped by the status quo, so that no real change is produced. But if the monkey wrench is big enough—if the disturbance is strong enough—the system simply can't absorb the shock. Unable to absorb the shock, the whole structure is forced to undergo a systemic change.

The mounting consequences of a chronic lack of taking proper care of ourselves can certainly be a monkey wrench of sufficient proportions to produce the systemic change that eventually restores balance, health and wholeness to our disordered lives. It is not too far a stretch to envision our sovereign Lord using a big monkey wrench of grace as He works all things together to bring about balance and harmony!

Perhaps that is why so many of us must undergo an emotional, physical, mental or spiritual "train wreck" before we are willing to begin doing everything just as the Lord has commanded! When small nudges fail, our gracious, loving Master applies greater and greater consequences—bigger and bigger monkey wrenches—until the consequences of our disordered lives finally drive us to our knees and into submission to His desire that we care for ourselves because of His great love for us.

Psalm 81:11-14 is a heartfelt plea from a loving, patient God to His stubborn, hardheaded people. Take time to read the Lord's simple instructions to you found in that passage of Scripture. (You might even want to substitute your name for the name "Israel.") After reading this passage, what word from God, if any, might you be ignoring that may result in a bigger monkey wrench instead of abundant blessing?

Psalm 81:16 states that those who listen to the Master are fed with the finest of wheat. With "honey from the rock," He satisfies His faithful ones. What will your decisions produce today: honey from a rock or a bigger monkey wrench? Why?

Lord, when I listen to Your voice and obey Your Word, You subdue my foes and bring me to a place of safety (see Psalm 81:13-14). Gracious Redeemer, I do want to be fed with the finest of wheat and honey from the rock. Today I will follow the path You have set before me (see Psalm 81:16). Amen.

Group Prayer Requests

4 first place
health

Today's Date: _____

Name	Request

Results

_____

_____

_____

_____

_____

_____

hope
perseveres

SCRIPTURE MEMORY VERSE

*Let us hold unswervingly to the hope we possess,
for he who promised is faithful.*

HEBREWS 10:23

During our Week Six lesson, we looked at the stories of men and women of faith who God graciously included in His Word as living examples of faith in action—faith that pleases Him. These ancients were commended for their faith; a faith that was sure of what they hoped for and certain of what they could not see. Summarize what you learned about action that supports our words of faith.

_____

_____

_____

_____

Turn to Hebrews 12:1. The faithful saints who have gone before us make a specific contribution to our journey today. What does it mean when the author states that we are "surrounded by such a great cloud of witnesses"?

_____

_____

_____

_____

By looking at their examples and learning from them, Hebrews 12:1 tells us we are encouraged to do two things. One is to throw off everything that _____ and the sin that ____ _____ _____. The second is to run with _____ the _____ marked out for _____. What is the race marked out for you in the First Place 4 Health program?

_____

_____

_____

_____

Day 1

WE POSSESS UNSWERVING HOPE

O gracious and loving Lord, as I study the different facets of hope, help me to understand why my hope in the past may have resulted in disappointment.

As we have worked our way through this Bible study, we have seen that hope takes on many facets. Listed below are some of the facets of hope we have learned about in previous lessons. Beside each type of hope, write a brief description of that specific aspect of hope.

Aspect of hope	Description of this aspect of hope
Deferred hope	
Expectant hope	
Living hope	
Joyful hope	

Aspect of hope	Description of this aspect of hope
Active hope	
Faith-filled hope	
Knowledgeable hope	
Obedient hope	

Our memory verse for the week tells us about another kind of hope. Look up the word "unswerving" in a dictionary and write the definition below.

_____

_____

_____

How is unswerving hope akin to running with perseverance?

_____

_____

_____

In the box under "Obedient hope" write "Persevering hope." Later, we will come back and write a brief explanation of what persevering hope looks like.

God, thank You for teaching me what genuine faith looks like. My faith is not founded in fleeting feelings but on the foundation of Your faithfulness. Amen.

PERSEVERANCE BEGINS WITH SELF-CONTROL

Thank You, Sovereign Lord, for servants like the apostle Peter who wrote down words to stimulate me to wholesome thinking and to remind me of Your will and way. Amen.

In an earlier session, we studied the words of 2 Peter 1:5-7. In this passage, the apostle Peter teaches us about the progression of our faith. He also teaches us that we are to obtain these aspects of faith in increasing measure. Why do you think attaining the elements of our faith in an orderly progression is important to our spiritual growth?

_____

_____

_____

_____

_____

How can we apply both step-by-step learning and the "increasing measure" principle to our First Place 4 Health efforts?

_____

_____

_____

_____

_____

In 2 Peter 3:1-2, Peter tells his good friends two reasons why he has written to them. What are those reasons?

1. _____

2. _____

Being stimulated to wholesome thinking and recalling the words spoken in the past will not lead to persevering faith if we are lacking one essential element. Look at the list of qualities Peter gives us in 2 Peter 1:5-7.

Notice that the quality of "self-control" comes between knowledge and perseverance. Perseverance can be described as long obedience in the same direction. But without self-control, what will we do?

_____

_____

_____

_____

First Peter 4:7 gives us another exhortation to be self-controlled. What two qualities allow us to be faithful in prayer?

1. _____
2. _____

James gives us an accurate description of what our path looks like when we lack self-control. What example does he use in James 1:6?

_____

_____

_____

_____

In James 1:8, what two words does James use to describe this person?

1. _____
2. _____

If you were to look at your First Place 4 Health efforts to date, which terms would best describe your path: "double-minded and unstable" or "unswerving in your faith"? Explain your answer.

_____

_____

_____

_____

More important than what your journey has looked like in the past, what is keeping you from being self-controlled and alert so that your path from this day forward will be one of renewed, persevering hope? Be specific.

_____

_____

_____

Forgive me, merciful Father, for those times when I have not been steadfast and unswerving in my devotion to You and to caring for myself as You ask. Today I praise You for Your incredible mercy and grace. Amen.

Day 3 — WE CAN RUN THE GOOD RACE

Gracious God, thank You that You never allow any temptation to overcome me, even the temptation to please others rather than You. Amen.

Our ability to persevere in hope, even when the path is rocky and we can't see the road beyond our immediate view, is determined by many things. One of those things is self-control. Yet there are often outside forces that influence our ability to stay on track. Paul, in writing to the Galatians, asked them an important question. After reading Galatians 5:7, write the question below.

_____

_____

_____

_____

Most of us begin a new diet-and-exercise program with great enthusiasm. We buy the books, we study the material, we plan healthy meals and exercise on a daily basis. And then one day, something happens. Just as we are lacing up our walking shoes to head out the door, someone or something else needs our time and attention. Looking back at Paul's words that you wrote above, what has just happened?

_____

_____

_____

_____

_____

Think of a time in the past week when an outside force cut in on your health and fitness goals. Describe the incident and your reaction.

_____

_____

_____

_____

Paul told the Philippians that he had let go of his past so that he could run the race set before him (see Philippians 3:13-15). Hebrews 12:1 tells us there are two other things we must let go of if we are going to run with perseverance. Write those two things below:

Throw off _____ that hinders and the _____ that so _____ entangles.

When you let other people and events interfere with your commitment to healthy living, what is the sin that easily entangles you? (Acts 5:29 tells you what you are not doing!)

_____

_____

_____

_____

What is the phrase we use for those who would rather please others than please God?

_____

_____

_____

_____

_____

Thank You, Father, for always giving me a way out when the temptation to be a people-pleaser comes my way. Amen.

Day 4 — GOD IS WITH US

O Lord God, You have promised to never leave me nor forsake me; that You will be with me until the end of the age. With You by my side, I cannot fail (see Joshua 1:5). Amen.

If we had to persevere along the road that leads to health and fitness in our own strength and power, the battle would be lost before we took the first step! But we do not have to make this journey on our own.

When the children of Israel were about to cross the Jordan River and enter the Promised Land, God told them they would not make this journey alone. Today we will use the words God gave Joshua and the Israelites as words of strength and encouragement for our journey too.

In Joshua 1:1 we learn that an important event had just happened. What had taken place that could have thrown the children of Israel off their appointed course?

_____

_____

_____

_____

_____

God had already appointed another leader to take the Israelites into the Promised Land. Read Joshua 1:1-5 to discover (1) the name and qualifications of the man God had appointed to lead the people, and (2) the assurance God gave His people so that they would not fall into doubt and fear. Record your findings.

_____

_____

_____

_____

What is the great and precious promise contained in the last sentence of verse 5?

_____

_____

_____

How are these words affirmed in Jesus' final words to His disciples before He ascended into heaven (see Matthew 28:20)?

_____

_____

_____

_____

Joshua 1:6 begins with a phrase that is repeated over and over again throughout the book of Joshua. What is that phrase?

_____

_____

_____

What else did God tell the Israelites to do in Joshua 1:7-9?

_____

_____

_____

_____

_____

Which will you choose to do today: Will you be strong, courageous and obedient, or will you allow yourself to be thrown off course? Explain your answer.

_____

_____

_____

_____

_____

Today, merciful Father, I pray that when I step out in strength and courage, I will never forget that obedience to Your commands is also part of my journey to health and wholeness. Amen.

Day 5 — GOD IS FAITHFUL

O Lord God, I thank You that Your ways are loving and faithful for those who keep the demands of Your covenant (see Psalm 25:10).

The memory verse for this week speaks of God's faithfulness. Write the verse below (from memory, if possible), and then explain how God's faithfulness is part of hope that perseveres.

_____

_____

_____

_____

_____

In 2 Peter 1:4, Peter not only tells us God's promises are very great and precious, but he also tells us the benefit they have in our lives. What does Peter tell us we can do through them?

How is participating in the divine nature and escaping the corruption in the world part of hope that perseveres?

In 1 Corinthians 10:13, the apostle Paul gives us an aspect of God's faithfulness that is essential to our ability to persevere. What is that aspect and why is it a necessary ingredient in perseverance?

How might God's great and precious promises be part of the means of escape He provides for us when we are under temptation?

In what ways is God's promise to never leave us or forsake us part of His faithfulness?

Proverbs 4:18-19 gives us valuable information about the path of the righteous—and the path of those who do not follow God's will and way. What is the path of the righteous like? What is the path of the wicked like?

_____

_____

_____

_____

How is a path that grows brighter every day part of the hope-in-action that allows you to persevere in a program such as First Place 4 Health?

_____

_____

_____

_____

Now that you have learned about persevering faith, go back to the Day 1 lesson and write what you have learned next to "Persevering hope." Aren't you glad that the God of hope is your constant companion and guide? Thank Him for His faithfulness now! You might want to record your prayer in your journal so that it becomes part of your faith-in-action story.

Sovereign Lord, I am so grateful that You are faithful to all Your promises and loving toward all that You have made (see Psalm 145:13). Amen.

Day 6

REFLECTION AND APPLICATION

O Lord, our Lord, how majestic is Your name in all the earth! You have set Your glory above the heavens (see Psalm 8:1). I will praise You, O Lord, with all my heart. Amen.

Hebrews 11:3 affirms that "by faith we understand that the universe was formed at God's command, so that what is seen was not made out of what was visible." Today in our reflection time, we are going to travel back in time to the beginning. Genesis 1:1 through Genesis 2:1 tells the marvelous creation story.

Turn to that passage and read it now. As you read, imagine that you are present, witnessing God's might and power as He speaks a word and it takes form and shape before your very eyes. Allow yourself to feel the wonder and awe of this account. See the stars burst forth. Watch the plants spring into a green carpet that covers the land. See the trees laden with seed-bearing fruit. Experience the animals as they receive breath and take their first steps.

When you have finished your meditation, conclude your reflection time by writing a prayer below or in your journal to the God of creation, thanking Him that He has created you and placed you in His wonderful world!

_____

_____

_____

_____

_____

Sovereign Creator, words cannot begin to express the wonder and awe I feel when I contemplate Your creation. Thank You for allowing me to be part of the creation You brought forth from nothingness. Amen.

REFLECTION AND APPLICATION Day 7

God of Hope, thank You for illuminating the things that have caused me to stumble in the past so that I will not repeat those same mistakes in the future. Today, Lord, I will pay attention to what You say. Amen.

This week we have learned about another important aspect of renewed hope: perseverance—being unswerving in our commitment to health and fitness as we run the race set before us. Write this week's memory verse from memory to affirm the reason you are able to persevere with hope.

_____

_____

_____

_____

_____

Our path to taking care of ourselves is not always one that grows brighter every day. We have hills and valleys on our journey—times when we cannot see the sun, let alone move forward at a rapid pace. And if our own internal attitudes weren't enough to keep us from attaining our goals, there are outside forces that cut in and keep us from running the path set before us. We make poor choices because pleasing God is not our first priority. We let others hinder our progress, often to the point of being so entangled that we lose our hope and vision.

Remember the poignant question the apostle Paul asked the Galatians: "You were running a good race. Who cut in on you and kept you from obeying the truth?" (Galatians 5:7). Today in your reflection time, ask yourself the same question.

Next, take a piece of paper and draw a road map of your journey toward health and wholeness that honors God. Each time you have swerved off the path, write a brief description of the person, event, place or thing that cut in on your progress. Be sure to begin your map on the day the Lord first laid it on your heart to honor Him by caring for your body as His holy temple. Continue the map of your journey until it reflects where you are today. You may need more than one sheet of paper to complete this exercise!

Once you have completed your road map, complete with notations about the pitfalls you have encountered along the way, go back and add *Caution* or *Stop* signs at each juncture where you lost your footing and swerved off course. Allow these notations to be red-flag warnings that will be part of the path you travel from this day forward. Part of renewing hope is learning from our mistakes! Knowing what went wrong allows us to throw off the sins that have hindered us so that we can walk on the straight path that leads to our health and fitness goals.

Loving Father, Your commandments are a lamp for my feet, and Your teaching is a light for my path. I know that the path You set before me is the way to life (see Proverbs 6:23). Thank You for the gift of hope. Amen.

Group Prayer Requests

4 first place
health

Today's Date: _____

Name	Request

Results

_____

_____

_____

_____

_____

_____

hope does not disappoint

SCRIPTURE MEMORY VERSE
*And hope does not disappoint us,
because God has poured out his love into our hearts
by the Holy Spirit, whom he has given us.*
ROMANS 5:5

There are two kinds of hope: *deferred hope* that makes our heart sick and *Spirit-filled hope* that does not disappoint us. Which kind of hope we reap depends on the daily choices we make—either we take the necessary action steps that make our hopes and dreams become reality or the passive route that leads to disappointment, disillusionment and despair.

The book of Proverbs often presents us with truth in a whimsical way by using characters that epitomize a way of life. Dame Folly is a loud, boastful person who talks a game she does not play. Lady Wisdom makes careful plans and diligently carries them out. The Simpleton represents an uneducated youth, someone lacking knowledge and understanding. The Fool does not acknowledge God or give thought to His ways. The Ant is industrious, and the Sluggard is lazy.

Turn to Proverbs 13:4. What do you learn about the difference between the Sluggard and the diligent Ant in this verse?

Now read Proverbs 20:4. What else do you learn about the Sluggard?

_____

_____

_____

_____

How do we resemble the Sluggard if we say we want to reap a bountiful crop when it comes to a healthy, balanced lifestyle, but we neglect to do the necessary work that will allow us to do so?

_____

_____

_____

_____

Let's look at one more proverb that talks about the Sluggard's fate. What does Proverbs 24:30-34 tell us the Sluggard has been doing instead of taking persistent action?

_____

_____

_____

_____

What is the result of his failure to take action? (Draw your answers from Proverbs 24:31.)

_____

_____

_____

_____

_____

As you go through this week's study, think about whether there is anything you are putting off until later that needs to be done today.

GOD GIVES US HOPE Day 1

Thank You, Lord, for Your Word and for giving me truth I can apply to my life through the whimsical characters portrayed in the book of Proverbs. Amen.

This week's memory verse explains the reason why hope will not disappoint us. The word "because" is the key to understanding this verse: Hope does not disappoint us because God has poured out His love into our hearts. Now look up the word "disappoint" in a dictionary. You will probably find more than one meaning given, so write down the various meanings of the word.

After carefully considering the meaning of "disappoint," answer the following questions as they apply to your First Place 4 Health efforts prior to working through this study.

Were you expecting something that did not materialize? If so, what were you expecting?

Were you left unsatisfied? If so, how?

Were your plans undone or frustrated? Explain.

_____

_____

_____

_____

If the Sluggard we read about in today's introduction came to you for advice, what would you tell him he needs to change to reap a bountiful harvest?

_____

_____

_____

_____

If deferred hope has been part of your First Place 4 Health story, how might the advice you just gave the Sluggard help you realize your health and fitness goals?

_____

_____

_____

_____

Gracious God, thank You for inviting me to leave my past behind so that I can press on toward the goal You have appointed for me. Amen.

Day 2 — GOD POURS OUT HIS LOVE

Today I kneel before You, Father, Son and Holy Spirit, asking that You empower me to care for my body, Your earthly temple, in a way that brings glory and honor to You. Amen.

When we are disappointed, our hopes and dreams are deflated, much like a bright, shiny balloon that has had the air let out of it! But our gracious God is not a God who lets us down. To the contrary, He builds us up by pouring His love into our hearts. How does God pour His love into us?

_____

_____

_____

_____

_____

_____

The apostle Paul told young Timothy three important things that the Spirit brings with Him when He takes up residence in our heart. Turn to 2 Timothy 1:7 and list those three things:

1. _____

2. _____

3. _____

What kind of spirit did God *not* give us?

_____

_____

_____

_____

_____

How is power part of a balanced program of health that honors God?

_____

_____

_____

_____

_____

The apostle Paul tells us that our body is the temple of the Holy Spirit, not just a humble home. Turn to 1 Corinthians 3:16 and 6:19. What do these verses tell you about this temple?

_____

_____

_____

_____

After having compared our bodies to temples in 1 Corinthians, Paul uses another analogy in 2 Corinthians 4:7. What does Paul compare our bodies to in this verse?

_____

_____

_____

What does the fact that our bodies are like jars of clay allow God to do?

_____

_____

_____

Does the way you care for yourself allow God's all-surpassing power to be displayed in you? Why or why not?

_____

_____

_____

_____

God, I am Your temple and Your Spirit lives in me. Help me to honor Your presence by caring for myself as a reflection of Your great love for me. Amen.

KNOWLEDGE GIVES HOPE

Day 3

O Lord God Almighty, Your love does surpass all knowledge, yet the more I grasp the magnitude of Your love, the more I am built up in my faith. Thank You for this incredible gift of Your love. Amen.

Read Paul's beautiful prayer for the saints found in Ephesians 3:14-21. Even though the prayer was offered for the believers living in Ephesus during the first century, it is also Paul's prayer for us who are living in the twenty-first century. Read Paul's words as you would read a prayer offered on your behalf, and make it your prayer.

Before whom is Paul kneeling when he offers this prayer, and how does Paul describe this person (see vv. 14-15)?

_____

_____

_____

How are Paul's words akin to the words Jesus taught His disciples when He told them to pray, "Our Father in heaven, hallowed be your name" (Matthew 6:9)?

_____

_____

_____

_____

In this prayer, Paul talks about the source of our power. Where does our power come from, and where does the source of it reside (see v. 16)?

_____

_____

_____

How does this affirm what we learned in our lesson yesterday?

_____

_____

_____

_____

In verse 17, Paul prays that we may be rooted and established in love. Reflecting back on last week's lessons, if we are not rooted and established in love, what do we resemble (see James 1:6-8)?

_____

_____

_____

_____

According to Ephesians 3:18, what does being rooted and established in love give us the power to do?

_____

_____

_____

_____

Paul continues his prayer by affirming that God is able to do immeasurably more than all we ask or imagine. How does God accomplish these wonderful things (see v. 20)?

_____

_____

_____

_____

There is a powerful benediction at the end of Paul's prayer. Write Ephesians 3:21 in the space below and then continue in prayer as you praise God for His power at work within you!

_____

_____

_____

_____

Gracious and loving Lord, You are able to do immeasurably more than I can ask, or even imagine, by the power of Your Spirit living and working within me (see Ephesians 3:20). Thank You for this assurance in Your Word. Amen.

GOD'S LOVE RENEWS HOPE   Day 4

O Father, help me to not just say I love You but also to extend Your love to my brothers and sisters in Christ—and to myself, as well. Amen.

During this week's study, we looked at three of the things the Spirit brings when He takes up residence in our heart. Unlike the spiritual gifts the Spirit brings, which vary from believer to believer as God chooses to distribute them, the three things Paul wrote to Timothy about are the birthright of all believers. What are those three things (see 2 Timothy 1:7)?

1. _____

2. _____

3. _____

Although we could study God's power, available to us through the Holy Spirit, for many lessons without exhausting the riches of this truth, today we will look at the second item on our list: love. The love spoken of here is not God's love for us, but our love for God and others. Yet love is not something that comes naturally to us. As human beings—jars of clay—how are we able to love? Turn to 1 John 4:19 and write the source of our love.

_____

_____

_____

_____

_____

Earlier in that same chapter, John tells us more about this love that comes from God (see 1 John 4:7-12). As you read the words, once again note that one of the apostles is addressing you as a dear friend. According to John, where does love come from (see v. 7)?

_____

_____

_____

_____

What do verses 7 and 8 tell us about the connection between knowing God's love and having the ability to love?

_____

_____

_____

_____

How did God show His love for us, and what is the end result of God's love as it is explained in verse 9?

_____

_____

_____

_____

First John 4:10 tells us that God loved us and sent His Son as an
_____ sacrifice for our sins. How does the fact that Jesus became
a sacrifice for our sins give us hope?

_____

_____

_____

_____

_____

_____

What is the end result of God's love for us, as given in verse 11?

_____

_____

_____

_____

_____

When we love each other, what happens (see v. 12)?

_____

_____

_____

_____

_____

How do you show love for God and for your brothers and sisters in
Christ? Give this question careful thought and write your response in
your journal.

Gracious and loving God, I can only love because You first loved me.
I know that I am in You and You are in me because You have given me
Your Spirit (see 1 John 4:13). Amen.

Day 5 GOD GIVES US SELF-DISCIPLINE

Wonderful Father, thank You for sending Your Holy Spirit to guide me into all truth. Your Word is truth; therefore, I will study Your Word in order to become more disciplined in my Christian life. Amen.

This week's memory verse, Romans 5:5, tells us that "_____ does not _____ us, because _____ has _____ out his _____ into our _____ by the _____ _____, whom ___ has _____ us." Reflect on what you have learned this week about this wonderful gift that God has given us. How is the Spirit's presence a reason for renewed hope?

_____
_____
_____
_____

We have power and the ability to love because God has poured His Spirit into our hearts! But there is one more aspect of the Spirit that was given in 2 Timothy 1:7; something we might not immediately consider a gift. What is that one thing?

_____
_____
_____

Although we may think of self-discipline and self-control as synonymous, they are not the same thing. Look up the words "discipline" and "control" in a dictionary and write the definitions you find.

Discipline:

_____
_____
_____

Control:

_____

_____

_____

What did you learn about the difference between self-discipline and self-control?

_____

_____

_____

_____

_____

Why are both self-discipline and self-control an integral part of renewed hope? Why are they an integral part of the First Place 4 Health program?

_____

_____

_____

_____

_____

How is spending time in God's Word and prayer part of our responsibility as disciples who want to learn how to be self-controlled?

_____

_____

_____

_____

In John 14:26, Jesus says, "But the Counselor, the Holy Spirit, whom the Father will send in my name, will teach you all things and will remind you of everything I have said to you." Not only does the Spirit teach us all truth, but He also gives us the desire—and the power—to apply that truth to our lives! How is Spirit-filled hope different from the deferred hope we learned about at the beginning of this study?

_____

_____

_____

_____

In Galatians 5:25, the apostle Paul tells us to "_____ in _____ with the _____." How will doing this not disappoint us as we move steadily toward our First Place 4 Health goals?

_____

_____

_____

_____

Sovereign Lord, help me manifest the fruit of self-control in my life so that my hope will not be deferred. Amen.

Day 6

REFLECTION AND APPLICATION

Thank You, loving Lord, for giving me the fruit of self-control so that I can exhibit the other fruit of the Spirit in abundant profusion that honors You.

During a recent women's gathering at a local church, one of the ladies described how she was redecorating her kitchen. She had replaced the floor with imported tile, purchased all new appliances, put up new window coverings and painted and wallpapered the walls. In keeping with her new décor, she had hired an artist-calligrapher to paint the fruit of the Spirit, as described in Galatians 5:22-23, around the ceiling board in vibrant colors that coordinated with her bright new color scheme. She then laughed and said, "All the fruit, that is, except self-control. Self-control isn't something we practice in the kitchen!"

Those of us who are striving to replace our destructive eating habits with prudent eating that honors God have learned that the kitchen is the first place in our home where we must diligently exercise self-control. No matter how much we want to be loving, joyful, at peace, patient with self and others, able to show kindness, goodness or gentleness—until we can put the fruit of self-control in place, all our other efforts will fail to produce abundant fruit. Without self-control, hope is nothing more than wishful thinking!

Like it or not, self-control is the fruit that allows us to display the other fruit of the Spirit so that others can see God's Spirit at work in our lives. Until self-control is in place, all the other Christian virtues outlined by the apostle Paul are just fancy words written on a page. Self-control is the virtue that allows us to grow our soul-garden and produce fruit that will grace every room in our homes—especially our kitchens.

How can you make a generous helping of self-control the ingredient that allows you to be self-controlled in your other healthy food choices?

_____

_____

_____

_____

How is self-control part of Spirit-filled hope? Think of the Sluggard in the introduction to this week's study. What could have changed the Sluggard's wishful thinking into an abundant crop?

_____

_____

_____

Lord, help me to never waste the good gifts You have given me because I do not exercise loving self-control. O Lord, You are my only hope. Because I trust in You, I am confident that I will not be disappointed. Amen.

REFLECTION AND APPLICATION

Lord, Your Word tells us that love is patient (see 1 Corinthians 13:4). Help me, Lord, to be patient with my progress during the renewing-hope process.

In Galatians 5:22-23, the apostle Paul gives us a list he calls the fruit of the Spirit. All of these nine fruit are manifest in all those in whom the Spirit of God dwells through faith in Christ Jesus. Although many of us learned to recite this list from memory, we often have difficulty applying these Christian virtues in a way that results in self-control.

On the chart below, write the name of the nine fruit of the Spirit. In the column next to that fruit, write what color you think that fruit would be if it were an actual piece of fruit growing on a tree, and explain why you chose that color.

Name of the fruit	Color of the fruit	Why I chose this color

Now describe how each fruit can be part of the First Place 4 Health menu that will give you renewed hope.

Name of the fruit	How this fruit can be part of the First Place 4 Health menu

God of Hope, You fill me with peace and joy as I trust in You. Thank You for pouring Your love into my heart by sending me Your Holy Spirit (see Romans 5:5). Thank You that Your hope does not disappoint. Amen.

Group Prayer Requests

4 first place health

Today's Date: _____

Name	Request

Results

_____
_____
_____
_____
_____
_____

overflowing hope

SCRIPTURE MEMORY VERSE

*But as for me, I will always have hope;
I will praise you more and more.*

PSALM 71:14

If you have applied the lessons we have learned during the past ten weeks of our study, by now you are not just hopeful that things can change but are also overflowing with hope—and confident that this time you will achieve your health and fitness goals, no matter how long you were stuck in deferred hope that led to disillusionment and despair.

As you have seen throughout *The Power of Hope* Bible study, hope that is not based on God's will, as revealed in His Word, is false hope that will not bring lasting change. However, the minute we are ready to give up our faulty beliefs and become willing to take the steps necessary to break the downward cycle, God Himself guarantees our success! Not because of our own human ability to change, but because He is the God of creation and re-creation, the God of Hope who pours His love into us by the power of His Holy Spirit.

Psalm 84:11-12 is a wonderful reminder of the benefit of walking before God in honesty and integrity. Take a moment to read those assuring verses. So often we make God's direction punitive and complicated rather than taking all He says and does as an expression of His incredible love and grace. As Psalm 84:11 reminds us, the Lord does not withhold any good thing from those who show their love for Him by obeying His commands.

HOPE THAT LEADS TO PRAISE

Lord Almighty, we truly are blessed as we put our trust in You and step out in confident hope that You are the One guiding our steps and showering us with Your favor! Amen.

This week's memory verse gives us an important truth about overflowing hope: It results in praise. Not praise for our human accomplishments or ability, but praise to the God of Hope who has filled us with the power and self-control to do all He asks us to do. Philippians 4:13 is a verse many of us have committed to memory. If you can write the verse from memory, do so. If not, look it up in your Bible and write it below.

Sadly, this verse is all too often pulled out of context and used as part of a faulty belief system that produces false hope. What if the thing we are doing is outside of God's will? Could we use Philippians 4:13 as a positive affirmation if we were undertaking something that was harmful to our health and wellbeing? Explain your answer.

In the past, in what ways, if any, has incorrect use of God's Word been part of the hope that disappointed you—and did not result in praise and honor being given to God?

How is knowing God's infallible Word—so that you can properly apply His great and precious promises and heed His warnings—an essential part of renewing hope?

_____

_____

_____

_____

O Lord God Almighty, You are my sun and my shield. How blessed I
am that You give me Your Word so that I can walk uprightly before You
(see Psalm 84:11-12). Amen.

HOPE THAT REMAINS STEADFAST

Day 2

Lord, when I am afraid, I will stand firm knowing that when I trust
in You, You will fight for me (see Exodus 14:13-14). Amen.

When the children of Israel were being led out of the cruel bondage of Egypt, they encountered what appeared to be an insurmountable obstacle. Pharaoh's army was about to overtake them, and the Red Sea was in front of them. They could not outrun the Egyptian soldiers in their chariots, and they could not cross the sea. In our vernacular, they were between a rock and a hard place! Exodus 14:10-12 tells us the reaction of the Israelites. Read those verses and restate them in your own words.

_____

_____

_____

Have there been times during this study when you felt as though it would be easier to return to your old ways than to continue with the health and balance you are learning in First Place 4 Health? Write about the most recent time you felt that way, and whether you fell back into destructive habits or continued to trust in God—and why.

_____

_____

_____

_____

What did you learn from that experience that will help you stay on track the next time you are tempted to turn back to your old ways?

_____

_____

_____

_____

Moses gave the frightened Israelites some advice that will keep us steadfast when we are in need of renewed hope. Read Moses' words in Exodus 14:13-14. How can you apply these words to your First Place 4 Health efforts?

_____

_____

_____

_____

Most of us are familiar with what happened next. However, it is always good to reread Bible passages that show God's might and power. Take a few moments to read Exodus 14:15-31.

_____

_____

_____

_____

What aspect of God's great power do you see displayed in this passage of Scripture that will give you renewed hope the next time you find your hope waning?

_____

_____

_____

End today's lesson by spending time praising God for hearing your cries of distress and coming in might and power to deliver you.

Gracious and loving Lord, thank You for bringing me to a place of renewed hope. When I put my trust in You and do things Your way, I am never disappointed. Amen.

HOPE THAT GIVES WAY TO PRAISE

Day 3

Lord God Almighty, who is like You? You are mighty, O Lord, and Your faithfulness surrounds You (see Psalm 89:8). Amen.

Throughout salvation history, God's people have burst into songs of jubilant praise when they witnessed God's might and power displayed in amazing ways. Their hope and trust gave way to songs of deliverance—songs of praise to the God of Hope in whom they had put their trust. By studying these songs of deliverance and hope, we, too, can allow our hope to overflow in words of praise to the God who deserves all honor and glory for what He has done for us.

Yesterday, we saw God's might and power displayed as He saved the Israelites from the Egyptian army. When the Israelites had all gone across the sea on dry land, Moses and his sister Miriam led the people of God in a song of praise to their Deliverer. That song is recorded for our benefit in Exodus 15:1-21. Read these verses now, and if you are able to do so, stand up and read the words out loud in joyful praise to the God who is your deliverer too!

Exodus 15:11 asks a question that is really a bold affirmation. What three aspects of God's character do we see outlined in this verse?

1. _____

2. _____

3. _____

How can God's majestic holiness, awesome glory and wonder-working power be part of the renewed hope you have through following the path God has set before you in the First Place 4 Health program? As you write your answer, address each attribute of God separately.

Holiness

_____

_____

_____

Awesome glory

_____

_____

_____

Wonder-working power

_____

_____

_____

Exodus 15:13 affirms God's unfailing love. What does this verse speak of God doing as a manifestation of His unfailing love?

_____

_____

_____

_____

How has God's unfailing love led you? How has the Lord's strength been part of the guidance you are receiving through the First Place 4 Health program? Again, take each part separately, and give specific examples!

_____

_____

_____

_____

Miriam's song (recorded in verse 21) gives a specific reason that God is to be highly exalted. God has thrown the horse and its rider into the sea. The horse and rider represent the power of our enemies, regardless of what form those enemies take. List three enemies that still keep you in fear and despair:

1. _____

2. _____

3. _____

Our wonder-working God is willing to cast your enemies into the sea too! What steps do you need to walk in expectant hope and stand firm as you witness God's deliverance?

_____

_____

_____

End your study time today with a song of praise to the God who has done mighty things for you. Miriam took her tambourine and danced as she sang. If you would like to express your praise in movement and song, do so. If not, record your song of praise in your journal.

Mighty God, I am blessed because I have learned to acclaim You by walking in the light of Your presence (see Psalm 89:15). Amen.

Day
4

MORE AND MORE HOPE!

Lord, I thank and praise You that I am among those You have filled with good things as part of Your enduring mercy. Amen.

After years of waiting for the promised Messiah, God's people had all but abandoned hope. The Jewish leaders and teachers of the law had become as oppressive as Pharaoh and the Egyptians in Moses' day. Turn to Luke 11:37-54 to better understand what the people of God were enduring. After reading this passage, list the six oppressive things they were doing to the people God was pleased to call His own.

1. _____
2. _____
3. _____
4. _____
5. _____
6. _____

Into this spiritual darkness came Jesus! The Son of God came to earth in human flesh. He moved into our neighborhood to bring spiritual light. Turn to Isaiah 9:2-7 to read Isaiah's prophecy that found fulfillment in the birth of Jesus Christ. Which of Isaiah's descriptions of Jesus, the Light of the World, is the one you need most right now? Why?

_____
_____
_____
_____

Upon learning that she had been chosen to be God's handmaiden—the Mighty One's instrument to be the Christ-bearer—Mary, like Moses and Miriam, broke into a song of praise. Mary's song is often called the Magnificat because, in this beautiful song of praise, Mary's soul magnified the Lord. Read Mary's song of praise in Luke 1:46-55. After reading, ask yourself what humble estate God has seen in you, and how He has extended His mercy to you in your distress. Record your thoughts.

_____

_____

_____

_____

_____

_____

What does God do to those who are proud in their innermost thoughts (see v. 51)?

_____

_____

_____

_____

What does God do for the humble?

_____

_____

_____

_____

How is getting rid of pride and replacing it with a humility that depends on God for all good things part of the renewed hope you are experiencing in the First Place 4 Health way of life?

_____

_____

_____

_____

_____

What does God do for those who are hungry, while the rich go away empty (see v. 53)? (Remember, this is more than just physical hunger.)

_____

_____

_____

_____

Luke 1:54 tells us that God has remembered to be merciful. To whom has He remembered to be merciful?

_____

_____

_____

_____

As a child of God, a member of God's family, you are Abraham's descendant, and God will remember to be merciful to you too! Spend the rest of your quiet time today praising God for His tender mercies that never fail those who trust in God's salvation.

When I put my hope in Your unfailing love, O God, and do what You have asked me to do, I can be confident that I will never be disappointed. How blessed are those who believe everything that You have said will come to pass. Amen.

Day 5

HOPE THAT ECHOES THROUGH THE AGES

Lord, today I kneel before You and give You thanks and praise. I will take Your words to heart and put them into practice, for You are my God of hope, the One in whom I will never be disappointed. Amen.

Even as we are singing marvelous songs of praise to God while we are here on earth, the day is coming when we will be invited to join the chorus praising Him throughout eternity. While our life here on earth is made up of many lesser hopes, as Christ followers, our ultimate hope is the hope of spending eternity in heaven with God. All the praise we have offered to our God here on earth is merely a prelude to the praise we will offer when Jesus comes to take His faithful people home!

When Jesus told the Parable of the Talents, He taught His disciples a valuable lesson in faithfulness. Turn to Matthew 25:21 and write the words the master said to the faithful servant.

_____

_____

_____

_____

When we read this parable, we tend to focus so much on the prospect of sharing our Master's happiness that we overlook some important words:

You have been _____ with a _____ things; I will _____ you in _____ of _____ things.

As you conclude this study, take time to list the things Your Master has called you to be faithful in through what you have learned. By mentally reviewing each of our weekly studies, you will be able to compile your list. What are the "few things" we must be faithful in if we are to have renewed hope and achieve our health and fitness goals?

_____

_____

_____

_____

Once you have reached your goal weight and achieved renewed health and balance, does that mean you can relax and take it easy? No! There is no such thing as retirement in the kingdom of God! Our duties may change as we age, but we must always be mindful of our responsibility before God. There is also no such thing as retirement from practicing the principles you have learned in First Place 4 Health! Why do you think that statement is true?

_____

_____

_____

Renewing your hope is an ongoing commitment to do the things that build hope, the things we have learned about during our Bible study. Unlike the downward cycle that leads to deferred hope, disillusionment and disappointment, renewing hope is an upward spiral. Like the path of the righteous that grows brighter every day, our hope will grow brighter and brighter as we do the things that are pleasing to God, the One who perpetually does marvelous things for those who love Him and keep His commands.

> The LORD bless you and keep you; the LORD make his face shine upon you and be gracious to you; the LORD turn his face toward you and give you peace (Numbers 6:24-27).

> *I call to You, O Lord, every day; I spread out my hands to You, confident that You hear my cries and will respond in mercy (see Psalm 88:9). Amen.*

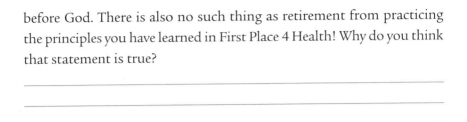

Day 6 — REFLECTION AND APPLICATION

God, You are compassionate and gracious, slow to anger, abounding in love. Thank You for Your goodness and grace to me (see Psalm 103:8). Amen.

As you have seen throughout our lessons, God's people have often used the psalms as the basis for their praise of God. Today we will do the same. Turn to Psalm 103, a psalm that focuses on God's benefits. We will use verses 3 through 6 to recap the benefits we have received from God as we have completed *The Power of Hope* Bible study:

Praise the Lord, O my soul;
all my inmost being, praise his holy name.
Praise the Lord, O my soul, and forget not all his benefits—
who forgives all your sins and heals all your diseases,
who redeems your life from the pit and crowns you with
love and compassion,
who satisfies your desires with good things so that your
youth is renewed like the eagle's.
The Lord works righteousness and justice for all the oppressed.

Reflect on verses 1 and 2. How is this a bold affirmation of the good things God has done for you—things that give you reason to praise God in the depths of your innermost being?

_____

_____

_____

For verses 3 to 6, describe how the particular benefit given in that verse is part of renewed hope through participation in First Place 4 Health.

Verse	Benefit
Psalm 103:3	
Psalm 103:4	
Psalm 103:5	
Psalm 103:6	

Lord, give me understanding, and I will keep Your law and obey it with all my heart (see Psalm 119:33-34). Teach me to do Your will, for You are my God. May Your Spirit lead me on level ground (see Psalm 143:10). Amen.

REFLECTION AND APPLICATION

Today, Lord, I will be still and know that You are God. You will be exalted in my life as I keep You first in all things (see Psalm 46:10). Amen.

We have come to the end of this Bible study, and next week your First Place 4 Health group will hold its victory celebration. Your faithfulness to follow your commitment to wholeness, balance and a healthy lifestyle that honors God gives you much to celebrate!

As you praise and thank God for the benefits you listed during your reflection time yesterday, remember that you are equipped to continue to do what you have learned. May you grow in grace and knowledge of the Lord Jesus Christ so that you can discover how to please Him in all you do, especially in the way you care for the body He created and entrusted to your safekeeping.

As part of your victory celebration, you will want to share with others what God has done for you during this 12-week renewing of hope journey. Take a moment to reflect on the lessons you have learned that have brought you to a place of renewed hope with regard to your balanced health. List four or five key things you have applied to your life—things that have made the biggest difference in your commitment to the precepts taught in the First Place 4 Health program. You may want to write your reflection in your journal to refer to when you need to be built up in your commitment to health, fitness and renewed hope.

May you continue to overflow with hope by the power of the Holy Spirit, because you live and move to the honor and glory of Jesus Christ your Lord!

Gracious God, You have poured out Your love into my heart. You have given me the Holy Spirit as my teacher, encourager and guide. Help me to hold unswervingly to the hope I possess, for You are always faithful! You are the One who strengthens me. Amen.

Group Prayer Requests

4health first place

Today's Date: _____

Name	Request

Results

_____

_____

_____

_____

_____

_____

time to celebrate!

To help shape your brief victory celebration testimony, work through the following questions in your prayer journal:

Day One: List some of the benefits you have gained by allowing the Lord to transform your life through this 12-week First Place 4 Health session. Be sure to list benefits you have received in the physical, mental, emotional and spiritual realms of your being.

Day Two: In what ways have you most significantly changed *mentally*? Have you seen a shift in the ways you think about yourself, food, your relationships or God? How has Scripture memory been a part of these shifts?

Day Three: In what ways have you most significantly changed *emotionally*? Have you begun to identify how your feelings influence your relationship to food and exercise? What are you doing to stay aware of your emotions, both positive and negative?

Day Four: In what ways have you most significantly changed *spiritually*? How has your relationship with God deepened? How has drawing closer to Him made a difference in the other three areas of your life?

Day Five: In what ways have you most significantly changed *physically*? Have you met or exceeded your weight/measurement goals? How has your health improved the past 12 weeks?

Day Six: Was there one person in your First Place 4 Health group who was particularly encouraging to you? How did their kindness make a difference in your First Place 4 Health journey?

Day Seven: Summarize the previous six questions into a one-page testimony, or "faith story," to share at your group's victory celebration.

May our gracious Lord bless and keep you as you continue to keep Him first in all things!

The Power of Hope
leader discussion guide

For in-depth information, guidance and helpful tips about leading a successful First Place 4 Health group, spend time studying the *First Place 4 Health Leader's Guide*. In it, you will find valuable answers to most of your questions as well as personal insights from many First Place 4 Health group leaders.

For the group meetings in this session, be sure to read and consider each week's discussion topics several days before the meeting—some questions and activities require supplies and/or planning to complete. Also, if you are leading a large group, plan to break into smaller groups for discussion and then come together as a large group to share your answers and responses. Make sure to appoint a capable leader for each small group so that discussions stay focused and on track (and be sure each group records their answers!).

week one: welcome to *The Power of Hope*

During this first week, welcome the members to your group, provide a brief overview of the First Place 4 Health program, explain what is expected of the participants at each of the weekly meetings, and collect the Member Surveys. (See the *First Place 4 Health Leader's Guide* for a detailed outline of how to conduct the first week's meeting.)

week two: heartsick and battle weary

Ask someone in your group who is committed to keeping a journal to talk about the benefits they have received from this practice. Then discuss what kinds of things members could record in their journals—prayers and praises, challenges, attitude shifts, victories, and more. Encourage everyone to start keeping a journal, but don't make it a guilt trip.

At the beginning of the Bible study portion of the meeting, have the group recite the words of Psalm 107:1, out loud and in unison.

Before the meeting, ask four group members to play the part of the on-the-spot news reporter covering each of the four groups of people in distress that we studied about during the week's studies.

Have each "roving reporter" give his or her on-the-spot account of what is happening, beginning with the person assigned to report on the people we read about. At the end of the report, have the rest of the group say, in unison, "Then they cried to the Lord in their distress and He saved them from their distress." Read what specific thing the Lord did for this group of people and lead a discussion about this action. Repeat for the other three days' lessons. At the end of all four reports, ask the group what the appropriate response of God's people is when He hears their cries for help and rescues them.

During the Day 6 reflection, members were asked to list the new things they learned about God from studying Psalm 107. Lead a group discussion about the various ways in which God revealed more about Himself through this study. Ask the group scribe to record the answers on a whiteboard or newsprint flip chart.

Ask the group how "fearless honesty" is part of crying out to the Lord, and how when they are not honest about what is happening in their life they cheat themselves out of God's assistance.

Lead a discussion about how crying out to the Lord in our distress is the beginning of renewed hope.

Ask the group what this week's lessons have taught them to heed and how they have found new ways to consider the great love of the Lord.

week three: put your hope in God

Begin your meeting with a discussion of David's qualifications to write Psalm 42. Ask group members what new things they learned about David during this week's lesson.

Most people, even long-time Christians, associate Psalm 23 with funeral and memorial services. Talk with your group about the "dark valleys" we experience other than the grief and sadness we feel when someone close to us dies. Relate the dark valley to the situation some in your group might have been in before coming to First Place 4 Health.

Before the meeting, ask someone to read the excerpt from the Phillip Keller book. After they have done so, read Psalm 139:1-6. Ask your group to talk about the plight of the "cast sheep," and the comfort they receive from the words of Psalm 139:1-6 when they are the sheep in danger.

It is important that the people in your group realize that God responds to our cries for help, not based on why we are in distress, but because of His great mercy. Be sure to emphasize that with your group. God does not take the "you made your bed, now lie in it" stance some of us are inclined to adopt!

First Place 4 Health is part of the soul care that keeps us from experiencing the spiritual dryness David talks about in Psalm 42. Ask members of your group to describe how the First Place 4 Health program, and the group they belong to, provides nourishment for their thirsty soul.

Read the beginning words of Psalm 42:5, "Why are you downcast, O my soul? Why so disturbed within me?" as though you were asking your group that question. Record the answers on a whiteboard or newsprint flip chart.

Talk to your group about how memorizing God's Word is part of the healthy self-talk that can be used to replace the negative tapes that keep us "downcast."

During the weeks ahead we will talk about many types of hope we can expect to experience as we travel from deferred hope to overflowing hope. Talk to the group about the three things we have done so far that are part of that transformation process. Put "Admitting the Truth of Our Condition," "Crying Out to God in Our Distress" and "Remembering God's Love and Faithfulness" on a whiteboard or newsprint flip chart and ask your group to talk about how these three things have been part of our renewing-hope journey in the first two weeks' lessons.

Be sensitive to the fact that some in your group may be suffering from clinical, not situational, depression. For them, medication is a necessary component of their recovery—but medication should always be combined with the truth of God's Word and the prescription the Great Physician has given us to deal with depression.

End your meeting with a prayer for all who suffer from a downcast soul and ask your group to encourage those who might be going through a dark valley right now and find themselves bearing a heavy burden.

week four: forgiveness renews hope

Before this meeting, be sure to spend time in prayer, asking God to give you the words to present the salvation message with truth and grace. Begin your lesson with the words of the prophet Jeremiah from the Day 1 study. Be sure that your group understands that whitewashing sin does not make it go away!

As part of the Day 7 Reflection, your group made a collage to symbolize the joy of new life in Christ. Display these during the meeting! Ask a member to read Isaiah 53. On a whiteboard or newsprint flip chart, ask the group to identify the four things Jesus carried to Calvary's cross.

Put the words "Substitutionary Atonement" on the whiteboard or chart. Lead a discussion about what these words mean. Perhaps you would like to divide the word "Atonement" into "At-one-ment," to signify that Jesus' atonement on our behalf is what allows us to be in relationship with God.

First John 1:5-10 talks about the importance of confessing our sins. After reading these verses, talk about the importance of confession—and what Scripture says we are doing when we claim to be without sin.

Ask if there are any sins God is not willing to forgive once we have confessed them to Him in earnest prayer. (If someone asks about the "unforgivable sin," answer by telling them that any sin we *believe* is unforgivable is the unforgivable sin, but if we believe God will forgive us when we confess our sins, there is nothing so horrible that God will not forgive us.)

Some of the people in your group may have been the victims of cruel abuse in their childhood. Some may be in abusive relationships even now. Be sure that they understand that forgiving an abuser is *not* saying what the abuser did was right. It is simply letting go of the resentment, bitterness or even hatred, so that the person can't continue to harm them through their remembrance of the abuse.

Talk about how a lack of confession or releasing bitterness through forgiving others is a great hindrance to progress in the First Place 4 Health program. Include some discussion of the concept of repentance (turning away from sin in a complete about-face).

Be sure to end the lesson with a declaration of forgiveness. You can use the last prayer from the Day 7 Reflection or one of your choosing, but do not omit this important means of grace.

week five: hope leads to action

Before the meeting, ask one or two members to share with the group about a time when they fell victim to the hope-without-action syndrome as it applies to participation in First Place 4 Health. Have them share their story at the beginning of the meeting.

Lead a discussion about how "wishing" is often disguised as "praying" in the Christian community. Invite group members to share their responses to the Lord's Prayer as it applies to your First Place 4 Health efforts. Have a group scribe record the responses on a whiteboard or newsprint flip chart.

The study also looked at some action we have already taken toward renewing hope. Because this action was about an attitude shift, it may not have felt like action to some in your group. Go through the list of things we have done, matching the action verb with the proper response.

Discuss how "going through the motions" is different from the joyful hope that leads to a genuine commitment to health and fitness goals.

Lead a discussion on how joyful hope, patient endurance and faithfulness in prayer work in tandem to bring balance and harmony to our lives. You may want to put the three actions on a whiteboard or flip chart and talk about how they form an upward cycle that leads to more and more hope.

Brainstorm with the group about how eliminating the people, places and things that put our First Place 4 Health program in jeopardy increases our joyful hope. Be sure to ask for specific examples of people, places and things your group members have identified as things they must eliminate if they are to succeed.

Split your group into 10 small groups (if you already have a small group, one person will be a group, or even, perhaps, say a word twice). Begin with group 1 and repeat the words of this week's memory verse with each group/person emphasizing a word (as in our Day 7 Reflection exercise). After you have done the exercise, talk to the larger group about what they have learned from this practice.

End the meeting with another time of reviewing the Lord's Prayer, but this time ask members to affirm the positive action they have taken to bring their words and actions into sync. Be sure to devote enough time to this exercise, as it makes our prayer life one of active faith rather than words without meaning.

week six: faith ensures hope

During this week's study we have looked at the "ancients," those people whose faith pleased God. Begin the meeting by talking about why their stories are an important part of our faith journey. (Romans 15:4 will guide your discussion.)

Ask group members about what they discovered when they looked up the words "certain," "sure" and "faith" in a thesaurus. Have a group scribe record the findings on a whiteboard or newsprint flip chart.

Noah did everything "just as the Lord told him." Lead a discussion about the significance of the word "just" in Noah's faith-in-action story. Be sure to emphasize that Noah did not know why he was doing things; he only knew he was to obey God.

In many ways our First Place 4 Health journey parallels Noah's story. Have the group talk about the elements in their journey that are certain and those that are not known.

Joseph gave the people certain instructions concerning his "bones." Talk about how these instructions were an act of faith, and what the group can learn from Joseph's faith in action.

The Ephesians burned their sorcery books so that they would not fall back into old habit patterns. Ask each group member to name one thing he or she needs to "burn" so that he or she doesn't look for a way back instead of looking forward with eyes of faith.

Ask the group what they learned from the story of Rahab. Have someone record the group's answers on a whiteboard or newsprint flip chart. Be sure to emphasize this woman of faith's place in salvation history!

Each person in your group will have researched one of the people of faith listed in Hebrews that we did not learn more about during this week's study. Allow time for members to present their findings. Be sure they emphasize what the person did that can be a lesson about faith in action we can use in the First Place 4 Health journey.

Conclude by discussing what is meant by the term "euphoric recall." Talk about how this might be undermining the participants' commitments to living a healthier lifestyle for God. Ask what the participants have learned from the men and women of faith they studied this week that will help them keep the past in the past.

week seven: knowledge increases hope

Have the group recite the words of Psalm 46:10 in unison.

With a member of the group acting as the recorder, review with your group what lessons they have learned about renewing their hope. Be sure to compile your own list before the meeting so you can stimulate their thoughts!

Ask your group how spending quiet time sitting at Jesus' feet and learning from Him is part of the renewing-hope process. Once again, have someone record the group's answers.

List the eight qualities we are to possess in increasing measure (see 2 Peter 1:5-7) on a whiteboard or newsprint flip chart. Talk about the way these attributes are arranged by Peter for our benefit.

Lead a group discussion about why knowledge comes before self-control and self-control comes before perseverance. Emphasize how each attribute prepares us to attain the next item on Peter's list.

Talk with the group about how their First Place 4 Health participation is like the fig tree planted in the vineyard owner's garden.

Jesus ends the Parable of the Persistent Widow with a very piercing question: "When the Son of Man comes, will he find faith on earth?" (Luke 18:8). Use this question to address how persistence in prayer is a necessary part of the First Place 4 Health program.

Your group went on two treasure hunts this week. One was a psalm-to-psalm treasure hunt looking for verses that show certain attributes of God, and the other was a nature walk looking for items that increase our knowledge of God by observing the world He created. Spend the rest of the meeting time allowing the group members to share the treasures that they found on these treasure hunts.

week eight: obedience builds hope

This week's memory verse asks a piercing question that all of us who call the name of Jesus must answer. Begin your meeting time by having the group recite this verse together in unison.

While we tend to think God's Word is difficult and complex, Scripture tells us otherwise. Have someone in your group read Deuteronomy 30:11-14, and then you lead a discussion of what these verses tell us about God's Word.

This week we looked at the life of Naaman, as found in 2 Kings 5:1-14. Before the meeting, ask one of your group members to be prepared to tell the story of Naaman as if he or she were an on-the-spot reporter covering these events. If you have a very creative group, you might consider having two or three members put on a skit.

All too often, we get angry at God and go off in a huff rather than accept His plan for our healing. Ask the group to share how they have been angry with God about some of the elements of the First Place 4 Health program and how that anger has kept them from obeying God's simple commands.

We looked at six attitudes that almost kept Naaman from receiving the Lord's healing. List the six attitudes on a whiteboard or newsprint flip chart. Have a member of the group act as the scribe to record answers. Go through each of the six attitudes, first identifying the part of Naaman's story that reveals this problem in Naaman, and then talking about how these six things can keep us from reaping the benefits of the First Place 4 Health program.

In large letters on your whiteboard or flip chart, write the word "problem." Talk about how Naaman's problem—leprosy—was the catalyst that allowed him to overcome the seven obstacles. Ask group members how the problem that brought them to First Place 4 Health can be a catalyst for healing in their lives too.

Works versus righteousness is a continual problem in the Christian community. Talk about how First Place 4 Health can be part of that counterproductive cycle of thinking that we can earn God's love.

Write "Bigger Monkey Wrench" on the whiteboard or flip chart, and talk about how a health or personal crisis can be the bigger monkey wrench that brings us to First Place 4 Health.

Conclude in prayer, asking God to use the challenges we face in our lives as a catalyst for change and as a means for drawing ourselves closer to Him.

week nine: hope perseveres

Have your group recite this week's memory verse in unison at the beginning of the meeting. Then you repeat the verse a couple more times, putting the emphasis on a different word each time. Talk about what new insight group members received by your using this technique.

Write the word "unswerving" on your whiteboard or newsprint flip chart. Ask your group to tell you what they learned about this word during this week's study.

This week we looked at the many facets of hope. Lead a discussion about these different facets of hope, and how, once we have gotten out of deferred hope, the other aspects of hope build on one another.

"Self-control" is not a word we particularly like, but it is a word that is necessary if we hope to persevere. Talk about why self-control must come before perseverance, and why knowledge comes before self-control.

Write the sentences, "You were running a good race. Who cut in and kept you from obeying the truth?" on your whiteboard or newsprint flip chart. Ask group members to share the things that cut in on their First Place 4 Health journey this past week.

Hebrews 12:1 tells us to let go of "everything that hinders." Talk about what the word "everything" entails.

The concept of God's faithfulness is important to our ability to persevere. Have some of the people in your group share their faithfulness verses with the entire group.

Write the words "I will never leave you nor forsake you" on your whiteboard or newsprint flip chart. Ask the group to explain how these words are an important part of their journey to renewed hope.

End your session with a prayer thanking God for His faithfulness and love.

week ten: hope does not disappoint

We can learn much from the wisdom of the proverbs, and the lessons the Sluggard has to teach us are especially valuable. Have your group talk about this slothful fellow. Why is deferred hope part of his life? How are we like him when we put off until tomorrow what we need to do today in First Place 4 Health?

Lead your group in a discussion about how disappointment is the result of not taking faith in action to support our hopes and expectations.

It is always God's desire to build us up in our faith. Put the three attributes of the Spirit that God has given us on your whiteboard or newsprint flip chart (see 2 Timothy 1:7). Ask three different members of your group to talk about each one, based on this week's lessons.

Ask someone in the group to share his or her thoughts on the two analogies the apostle Paul uses to describe our bodies: a temple and a jar of clay. Have that person focus on what each analogy allows God's glory to do in and through us.

Paul's prayer in Ephesians 3:16-21 is a beautiful example of the Trinity in action. Read this passage to your group and then lead a discussion about how the Father, Son and Holy Spirit all have a specific role to play in our salvation.

Put the words "self-discipline" and "self-control" on your whiteboard or newsprint flip chart. Ask the group to define each concept and talk about how they are alike and how they are different.

Ask your group why both self-discipline and self-control are necessary for success in their health journey.

Lead a discussion about how we walk in step with the Spirit.

The Day 7 Reflection was about the fruit of the Spirit. Have your group talk about what colors they chose for the various fruits and why. Ask them to identify how each fruit of the Spirit is part of their First Place 4 Health efforts.

End this session with Paul's benediction (see Ephesians 3:16-21) and make it your prayer for your group.

week eleven: overflowing hope

This week's lesson reminds us that overflowing hope results in praise to God. Read Psalm 84. Allow time for all members of your group to share words or phrases from the psalm that assure them of God's love and power.

Ask group members to share which old, unhealthy habits cause them to struggle the most. Why is it sometimes tempting to return to old habits rather than move toward the health and balance they are learning? What helps them stay on track?

Ask your group why the correct handling of God's Word is vital to a healthy relationship with God. Knowing God's Word helps us stay on track. The more we know His Word, the more confident we can be that our trust in Him is secure.

Discuss what attributes of God renew their hope and trust in Him. How do these attributes encourage them to persevere on the path God has set before them in the First Place 4 Health Program?

Write "Trust" on the left side, "Hope" in the middle and "Praise" on the right side of your whiteboard or newsprint flip chart. Draw an arrow from "Trust" to "Hope" to "Praise." Ask your group how trust in God leads to hope and then to praise. Allow time for group members to share experiences where they have made this connection between trust and praise.

Talk about some of the ways in which God responds to the humble (see Luke 1:46-56). How does replacing pride with humility renew a person's hope and lead to praise?

Ask the group members how, after they have met their goal weight, they plan to continue to practice the principles they have learned to keep their hope growing brighter.

Discuss what it means to praise God with your "inmost being." End your time together by reading Psalm 103. Ask group members to reflect on the good things that God has done for them as you read.

week twelve: time to celebrate!

Even though most of your meeting this week will be a victory celebration, take some time at the beginning of the meeting to talk about how much God loves each person in the group and that each of us is called to love our brothers and sisters in Christ. (See "Planning a Victory Celebration" in the *First Place 4 Health Leader's Guide* for ideas about throwing a successful celebration for your group.)

For the rest of the study time, allow each member to tell his or her *The Power of Hope* story. Give members an equal opportunity to share the goals they set for themselves at the beginning of the 12-week session and talk about the challenges and good things God has done for them throughout the process. Don't allow the more talkative group members to monopolize all the time. Even those who have not met their goals have still been part of the journey, so allow them to share and talk about their challenges and why they did not make their goals.

Making a commitment to continue in First Place 4 Health is an important part of victory. Be sure to talk about your group's future plans, and make each person feel welcome to continue the journey with you.

First Place 4 Health menu plans

Each menu plan is based on approximately 1,400 to 1,500 calories per day. All recipe and menu exchanges were determined using the Master-Cook software, a program that accesses a database containing more than 6,000 food items prepared using the United States Department of Agriculture (USDA) publications and information from food manufacturers. As with any nutritional program, MasterCook calculates the nutritional values of the recipes based on ingredients. Nutrition may vary due to how the food is prepared, where the food comes from, soil content, season, ripeness, processing and method of preparation. For these reasons, please use the recipes and menu plans as approximate guides. Consult a physician and/or a registered dietitian before starting a weight-loss program.

For those who need more calories, add the following to the 1,400-calorie plan:

- 1,800 calories: 2 ounce equivalent of meat, 3 ounce equivalent of bread, $^1/_2$ cup vegetable serving, 1 tsp. fat

- 2,000 calories: 2 ounce equivalent of meat, 4 ounce equivalent of bread, $^1/_2$ cup vegetable serving, 3 tsp. fat

- 2,200 calories: 2 ounce equivalent of meat, 5 ounce equivalent of bread, $^1/_2$ cup vegetable serving, $^1/_2$ cup fruit serving, 5 tsp. fat

- 2,400 calories: 2 ounce equivalent of meat, 6 ounce equivalent of bread, 1 cup vegetable serving, $^1/_2$ cup fruit serving, 6 tsp. fat

First Week Grocery List

Produce
☐ alfalfa sprouts
☐ apples
☐ baby carrots
☐ banana
☐ bean sprouts
☐ broccoli florets
☐ cantaloupe
☐ carrots
☐ celery
☐ cilantro
☐ coleslaw
☐ cucumbers
☐ garlic
☐ grapefruit
☐ grapes
☐ green bell pepper
☐ green onions
☐ jalapeño peppers
☐ Mandarin oranges
☐ melon
☐ mixed dark salad greens
☐ mushrooms
☐ onion
☐ orange
☐ parsley
☐ potatoes
☐ red bell pepper
☐ red onion
☐ red potatoes
☐ salad
☐ strawberries
☐ tomatoes
☐ zucchini

Baking Products
☐ all-fruit spread
☐ black pepper

☐ canola oil
☐ cooking sherry
☐ cornstarch
☐ Dijon mustard
☐ garlic, granulated
☐ lemon pepper seasoning
☐ lime juice
☐ lowfat dressing
☐ mayonnaise
☐ mixed berries
☐ nonstick cooking spray
☐ olive oil
☐ orange marmalade, reduced-sugar
☐ oriental sesame oil
☐ pepper
☐ raisins
☐ Ranch dressing
☐ red cooking wine
☐ red kidney beans
☐ rice wine vinegar
☐ salsa
☐ salt
☐ soy sauce, low-sodium
☐ spaghetti sauce
☐ tomato paste

Breads and Cereals
☐ Bran flakes cereal
☐ bread, whole-wheat
☐ breadsticks
☐ dinner rolls
☐ flour tortillas
☐ flat pita bread
☐ Grape Nuts® cereal
☐ grits
☐ linguine noodles
☐ penne pasta

- [ ] rotini pasta
- [ ] saltine crackers
- [ ] spaghetti sauce, chunky-style

Canned Foods
- [ ] beef broth, fat-free
- [ ] Campbell's® Chunky™ Minestrone Soup
- [ ] cut green beans
- [ ] tuna

Dairy Products
- [ ] apple juice
- [ ] cheddar cheese, lowfat
- [ ] eggs
- [ ] egg substitute
- [ ] margarine, reduced-calorie
- [ ] margarine, reduced-fat
- [ ] milk, nonfat
- [ ] mozzarella cheese, lowfat
- [ ] orange juice

- [ ] sour cream, reduced-fat
- [ ] whipped topping, nondairy
- [ ] yogurt, plain nonfat

Frozen Foods
- [ ] Healthy Choice® Glazed Chicken
- [ ] stir-fry vegetables

Meat and Poultry
- [ ] beef sirloin, lean
- [ ] chicken breasts, boneless and skinless
- [ ] chuck roast, lean and boneless
- [ ] fillet mignon
- [ ] ground beef, extra lean
- [ ] pork loin chops, boneless
- [ ] shrimp
- [ ] turkey bacon
- [ ] turkey pepperoni slices
- [ ] turkey sausage

First Week Meals and Recipes

DAY 1

Breakfast

(2) 6-in. low-fat flour tortillas
$^1/_2$ cup egg substitute
2 tbsp. chopped onion

2 tbsp. chopped bell pepper
2 tbsp. salsa
nonstick cooking spray

Scramble egg substitute, onion, bell pepper and salsa in skillet sprayed with nonstick cooking spray. Spoon $^1/_2$ cooked mixture into each tortilla and roll into burrito. Serve with 1 small orange. Serves 1.

Nutritional Information: 275 calories; 14g fat (43.5% calories from fat); 16g protein; 24g carbohydrate; 4g dietary fiber; 2mg cholesterol; 381mg sodium.

Lunch

Arby's® Junior Roast Beef Sandwich
1 cup coleslaw

1 cup mixed melon balls

Nutritional Information: 473 calories; 18g fat (31.5% calories from fat); 20g protein; 66g carbohydrate; 5g dietary fiber; 40mg cholesterol; 869mg sodium.

Dinner

2 cups salad, tossed with 2 tbsp. low-fat dressing
1 small (1 oz.) dinner roll, topped with 1 tsp. reduced-fat margarine

1 Healthy Choice® Glazed Chicken
$^3/_4$ cup fresh berries, topped with 1 tbsp. nondairy whipped topping

Nutritional Information: 493 calories; 14g fat (24.9% calories from fat); 20g protein; 72g carbohydrate; 12g dietary fiber; 32mg cholesterol; 1,071mg sodium.

DAY 2

Breakfast

$^1/_2$ cup cooked grits, topped with 1 tsp. reduced-fat margarine
1 small banana
1 cup nonfat milk

1 slice light whole-wheat bread, toasted and topped with 1 tsp. all-fruit spread

Nutritional Information: 546 calories; 3g fat (4.5% calories from fat); 19g protein; 115g carbohydrate; 6g dietary fiber; 4mg cholesterol; 253mg sodium.

....

Lunch
Turkey Pepperoni and Veggie Pizza

(1) 6-in. flat pita bread
$^{1}/_{4}$ cup prepared chunky-style
    spaghetti sauce
8 turkey pepperoni slices
$^{1}/_{4}$ cup shredded carrots

$^{1}/_{4}$ cup cooked broccoli florets
$^{1}/_{4}$ cup diced tomatoes
1 oz. low-fat mozzarella cheese,
    shredded

Preheat oven to 450° F. Place pita bread on cookie sheet and spread spaghetti sauce over bread. Layer with remaining ingredients, finishing with cheese. Bake 8 to 10 minutes or until cheese is melted. Serve with 1 small orange. Serves 1.

Nutritional Information: 410 calories; 15g fat (33.3% calories from fat); 19g protein; 50g carbohydrate; 5g dietary fiber; 30mg cholesterol; 1,050mg sodium.

....

Dinner
Beef Stir-Fry

1 lb. lean beef sirloin
2 tsp. canola oil
1 tsp. chopped garlic
4 oz. uncooked linguine noodles
1 small red onion, sliced
1 cup sliced carrots

1 cup diced zucchini
3 tbsp. water
1 cup fresh broccoli florets
1 cup sliced mushrooms
1 tsp. soy sauce
nonstick cooking spray

Heat oil over high heat in skillet sprayed with cooking spray. Add beef and garlic, and then stir-fry until cooked to your liking. Remove from skillet and keep warm. Cook noodles according to package directions, omitting salt and fat. Drain and keep warm. Stir-fry onion and carrots until carrots are partially done, adding water as needed to prevent sticking. Add zucchini, broccoli, mushrooms and soy sauce. (**Note:** Any combination of vegetables may be used.) Stir-fry until vegetables are done to your liking. Add beef to reheat, and then toss with pasta. Serve with a 1-ounce breadstick and 1 cup sliced strawberries topped with 1 tablespoon nondairy whipped topping. Serves 4.

Nutritional Information: 427 calories; 12g fat (24.7% calories from fat); 41g protein; 39g carbohydrate; 4g dietary fiber; 75mg cholesterol; 225mg sodium.

DAY 3

Breakfast

Turkey Bacon and Egg Sandwich

2 slices light whole-wheat bread, toasted and topped with 1 egg (cooked in a nonstick pan), 1 strip turkey bacon (cooked crisp)

Serve with 1 medium apple.

Nutritional Information: 281 calories; 9g fat (27.5% calories from fat); 13g protein; 42g carbohydrate; 9g dietary fiber; 224mg cholesterol; 489mg sodium.

Lunch

1 cup Campbell's® Chunky™   2 tomato slices
  Minestrone Soup $1/2$ cup baby carrots
6 saltine crackers   2 tbsp. low-fat Ranch dressing
1 cup mixed dark salad greens with $1/2$ cup apple juice

Nutritional Information: 260 calories; 9g fat (30.6% calories from fat); 4g protein; 42g carbohydrate; 4g dietary fiber; 0g cholesterol; 561mg sodium.

Dinner

Grilled Fillet Mignon

3-oz. fillet mignon per person, grilled to your liking

Serve each steak with $1/2$ cup steamed broccoli and a 6-ounce baked potato topped with 1 teaspoon reduced-fat margarine, 1 teaspoon salsa and 1 teaspoon reduced-fat sour cream. Serves 1.

Nutritional Information: 412 calories; 22g fat (48.5% calories from fat); 20g protein; 33g carbohydrate; 4g dietary fiber; 62mg cholesterol; 157mg sodium.

DAY 4

Breakfast

$1/4$ medium cantaloupe, topped with 1 cup plain nonfat yogurt, 2 tbsp. raisins and 1 tbsp. Grape Nuts® cereal

Nutritional Information: 255 calories; 1g fat (3.2% calories from fat); 16g protein; 49g carbohydrate; 3g dietary fiber; 4mg cholesterol; 238mg sodium.

Lunch

Tuna Salad Pita

(1) 7-in. whole-wheat pita, cut
   in half crosswise to form
   2 pockets
(1) 4-oz. can water-packed tuna,
   drained
$1/4$ cup chopped onion

$1/4$ cup chopped celery
2 tsp. low-fat mayonnaise
$1/4$ tsp. lemon-pepper
   seasoning
$1/2$ cup alfalfa sprouts

In small bowl, combine tuna, onion, celery, mayonnaise and lemon-pepper seasoning. Fill each pita pocket with half of tuna salad and top each with $1/4$ cup alfalfa sprouts. Serve with 1 cup cucumber rounds, 1 cup carrot sticks and 15 grapes. Serves 1.

Nutritional Information: 401 calories; 5g fat (10.1% calories from fat); 38g protein; 54g carbohydrate; 9g dietary fiber; 37mg cholesterol; 703mg sodium.

Dinner

Pasta Primavera with Meat Sauce

1 lb. extra-lean ground beef
6 oz. uncooked penne pasta
$1/4$ cup diced onion
$1/4$ cup diced red or green
   bell pepper
1 cup sliced mushrooms
1 tsp. granulated garlic

1 tsp. salt
3 cups prepared spaghetti sauce
(1) 10-oz. pkg. frozen stir-fry
   vegetables, thawed
nonstick cooking spray

Cook pasta according to package directions, omitting salt and fat. Drain and set aside. Sauté onion and bell pepper in a large saucepan coated with cooking spray. Add mushrooms, garlic, salt and ground beef. Cook for 12 minutes or until done. Drain off excess fat and add spaghetti sauce and vegetables. Simmer for 5 minutes more, and then serve over pasta. Serve with 1 cup green salad tossed with 2 tablespoons low-fat dressing and a 1-ounce breadstick. Serves 4.

Nutritional Information: 704 calories; 30g fat (38.8% calories from fat); 33g protein; 75g carbohydrate; 10g dietary fiber; 79mg cholesterol; 1,660mg sodium.

DAY 5

Breakfast

Brunch Casserole

4 slices whole-wheat bread, crusts removed
2 oz. low-fat turkey sausage
1/4 cup chopped mushrooms
1 tsp. chopped onion
3 eggs, beaten

1 cup nonfat milk
1/4 tsp. salt
1/8 tsp. black pepper
1/8 tsp. granulated garlic
2 oz. low-fat cheddar cheese, shredded

Line bottom of 9" x 9" casserole dish with bread. Sauté sausage in nonstick skillet until done. Remove sausage and sauté mushrooms and onions until tender. Crumble sausage and combine with mushrooms and onion, and then sprinkle mixture on top of bread. Combine eggs, milk, salt, pepper and garlic. Mix well and pour over sausage. Sprinkle with cheese, and then cover and refrigerate overnight. Set out for 15 minutes prior to baking, and then bake at 350° F for 40 to 45 minutes. Serve each with 1/2 grapefruit. Serves 4.

Nutritional Information: 215 calories; 9g fat (36.3% calories from fat); 15g protein; 19g carbohydrate; 2g dietary fiber; 174mg cholesterol; 547mg sodium.

Lunch

Oriental Seafood Pasta Salad

2 oz. (about 6 medium) cooked shrimp, peeled and deveined
1/2 cup cooked rotini pasta
1/2 cup bean sprouts
1/2 cup sliced celery

1/2 cup Mandarin oranges
1/4 cup cooked red kidney beans, drained
1 tbsp. rice wine vinegar
1/2 tsp. oriental sesame oil

Serve with 1/2 pita bread (toasted).

Nutritional Information: 441 calories; 4g fat (8.9% calories from fat); 26g protein; 75g carbohydrate; 9g dietary fiber; 111mg cholesterol; 348mg sodium.

Dinner

Hearty Vegetable and Beef Stew

3/4 lb. boneless, lean chuck roast, trimmed of fat, cut into 1/2-in. cubes

(2) 14 1/4-oz. cans fat-free beef broth
2 tsp. olive oil, divided

1 large onion, sliced
$^1/_3$ cup tomato paste
3 garlic cloves, minced
3 cups cubed carrots
3 cups cubed red potatoes
$2^1/_2$ cups quartered
   mushrooms

$^1/_2$ cup red cooking wine
$^1/_4$ tsp. pepper
(1) 8-oz. can cut green beans
2 tbsp. water
1 tbsp. cornstarch
chopped fresh parsley
   (optional)

In medium saucepan, bring beef broth to boil. Boil 15 minutes or until re-duced to 2 cups, and then remove from heat and set aside. In a large Dutch oven, heat 1 teaspoon oil over medium-high heat. Add beef, brown on one side, and remove from pan. Heat remaining oil in pan over medium-high heat, and then add onion, tomato paste and garlic. Cook for 5 minutes, stir-ring constantly. Return beef to pan, and then add reduced broth, carrots, po-tatoes, mushrooms, cooking wine, pepper and green beans. Bring to boil and then cover, reduce heat and simmer 45 minutes or until vegetables are tender. In small bowl, combine water and cornstarch. Stir well to remove lumps, and then add to the stew. Bring to a boil and cook for 1 minute, stir-ring constantly. Ladle 2 cups of stew into each soup bowl and garnish with parsley, if desired. Serve each with 1 cup salad with 2 tablespoons low-fat dressing. Serves 4.

Nutritional Information: 434 calories; 17g fat (33.7% calories from fat); 29g protein; 46g car-bohydrate; 8g dietary fiber; 50mg cholesterol; 906mg sodium.

DAY 6

Breakfast
McDonald's® Egg McMuffin®   6 oz. orange juice

Nutritional Information: 377 calories; 12g fat (29.3% calories from fat); 19g protein; 48g car-bohydrate; 2g dietary fiber; 260mg cholesterol; 822mg sodium.

Lunch
Chick-fil-A® Chargrilled Chicken   1 small carrot-and-raisin side salad
   Sandwich   15 red grapes

Nutritional Information: 477 calories; 9g fat (16.8% calories from fat); 28g protein; 74g car-bohydrate; 10g dietary fiber; 60mg cholesterol; 1,412mg sodium.

Dinner

Orange Pork Chops

(4) 4-oz. boneless pork loin chops
$^1/_3$ cup reduced-sugar orange
  marmalade
2 tbsp. Dijon mustard

1 bunch green onions, trimmed
2 cups Mandarin oranges
nonstick cooking spray

Preheat broiler or outdoor grill to high. In a small saucepan, combine marmalade and mustard. Heat to medium, stirring constantly until marmalade is melted, and then remove from heat and set aside. Drain juice from oranges and set fruit aside. Place chops on broiler pan. Broil chops about 4 inches from heat for 6 minutes, and then turn and broil 2 more minutes. Spoon half of marmalade glaze over chops, and continue broiling 3 to 4 minutes more or until chops are no longer pink. While meat is cooking, slice green onions diagonally into 1-inch pieces. Stir-fry in skillet coated with cooking spray for 2 minutes or until tender-crisp. Stir in remaining glaze until heated and add oranges; serve over chops. Serve each with $^3/_4$ cup potato salad and 1 cup assorted grilled vegetables. Serves 4.

Nutritional Information: 246 calories; 8g fat (30.9% calories from fat); 17g protein; 25g carbohydrate; 3g dietary fiber; 67mg cholesterol; 373mg sodium.

DAY 7

Breakfast

$^1/_2$ cup bran-flakes cereal
1 tbsp. raisins
1 cup nonfat milk

1 slice whole-wheat bread, toasted
and topped with 1 tsp. all-fruit
spread

Nutritional Information: 259 calories; 2g fat (6.3% calories from fat); 14g protein; 51g carbohydrate; 6g dietary fiber; 4mg cholesterol; 458mg sodium.

Lunch

6-in. Subway® Cold Cut Trio sandwich
  (no added fat or cheese), made with
  lots of veggies

1 cup mixed berries

Note: You may substitute 1 bag of baked potato chips for $^1/_2$ of the sandwich bread, if desired.

Nutritional Information: 325 calories; 12g fat (34% calories from fat); 10g protein; 48g carbohydrate; 5g dietary fiber; 20g cholesterol; 1,450mg sodium.

Dinner

Grilled Chicken Breasts with Corn Salsa

(4) 4-oz. boneless, skinless chicken
 breasts
$^1/_2$ cup cooking sherry
1 tbsp. low-sodium soy sauce
1 tbsp. chopped fresh cilantro

2 tsp. fresh lime juice
1 to 2 tsp. seeded and chopped
 jalapeño peppers
salt and pepper to taste

Combine sherry, soy sauce, cilantro, lime juice and jalapeños in medium bowl. Mix well; add chicken and turn to coat. Cover and marinate in refrigerator at least 1 hour, or up to 4 hours, turning occasionally. Preheat barbecue or broiler to medium-high. Remove chicken from marinade and discard liquid. Season chicken with salt and pepper and then grill or broil chicken until cooked through (about 4 minutes each side). Cut into thin diagonal slices and top each with Corn Salsa (see additional recipes section). Serve each with 1 cup cooked green beans mixed with a little salsa; 2 cups spinach salad with mushrooms, tomatoes and 2 tablespoons low-fat dressing; and a 1-ounce dinner roll with 1 teaspoon reduced-calorie margarine. Serves 4.

Nutritional Information: 352 calories; 6g fat (17.7% calories from fat); 32g protein; 35g carbohydrate; 5g dietary fiber; 66mg cholesterol; 476mg sodium.

Second Week Grocery List

Produce
- [ ] alfalfa sprouts
- [ ] apples
- [ ] blueberries
- [ ] broccoli
- [ ] butternut squash
- [ ] carrots
- [ ] celery
- [ ] eggplants
- [ ] garlic
- [ ] grapefruit
- [ ] grapes
- [ ] green bell peppers
- [ ] green onions
- [ ] lettuce
- [ ] lettuce, romaine
- [ ] mixed berries
- [ ] mushrooms
- [ ] onions
- [ ] oranges
- [ ] peaches
- [ ] potatoes
- [ ] raspberries
- [ ] red bell pepper
- [ ] red onions
- [ ] red potatoes
- [ ] salad
- [ ] spinach
- [ ] strawberries
- [ ] tomatoes

Baking Products
- [ ] all-purpose flour
- [ ] applesauce, unsweetened
- [ ] baking powder
- [ ] baking soda
- [ ] basil, dried
- [ ] black pepper, ground

- [ ] cayenne pepper
- [ ] chili powder
- [ ] cinnamon
- [ ] cumin, ground
- [ ] Dijon mustard
- [ ] garlic powder
- [ ] gelatin, sugar-free, white-grape flavored
- [ ] Italian dressing, lowfat
- [ ] lowfat dressing
- [ ] nonstick cooking spray
- [ ] nutmeg
- [ ] oatmeal
- [ ] olive oil
- [ ] onion powder
- [ ] paprika
- [ ] pepper
- [ ] raisins
- [ ] Ranch dressing, lowfat
- [ ] sage, dried rubbed
- [ ] salsa
- [ ] salt
- [ ] sugar
- [ ] sugar or Splenda® equivalent
- [ ] syrup, sugar-free
- [ ] Thousand Island dressing, lowfat
- [ ] vanilla extract
- [ ] walnuts
- [ ] Worcestershire sauce

Breads and Cereals
- [ ] bagels, whole-wheat
- [ ] bread, cinnamon-raisin
- [ ] bread, Italian or French
- [ ] bread, whole-wheat
- [ ] breadsticks

- ❑ corn tortillas
- ❑ crackers
- ❑ dinner roll, whole-wheat
- ❑ English muffins
- ❑ hoagie rolls with sesame seeds
- ❑ oyster crackers
- ❑ saltine crackers

Canned Foods
- ❑ black beans
- ❑ chicken broth, low-sodium
- ❑ corn
- ❑ great Northern beans
- ❑ kidney beans
- ❑ tomatoes, diced
- ❑ tomato sauce
- ❑ tomato soup, ready-to-eat
- ❑ vegetable soup, 90-calorie

Dairy Products
- ❑ butter
- ❑ buttermilk
- ❑ cheddar cheese, 2-percent
- ❑ cheddar cheese, reduced-fat
- ❑ cheddar cheese, reduced-fat and extra-sharp
- ❑ cream cheese, fat-free
- ❑ eggs
- ❑ egg substitute

- ❑ Gruyère cheese
- ❑ margarine, reduced-calorie
- ❑ mayonnaise, lowfat
- ❑ milk, fat-free
- ❑ milk, 1-percent lowfat
- ❑ milk, nonfat
- ❑ provolone cheese, reduced-fat
- ❑ sour cream, reduced-fat
- ❑ Swiss cheese, reduced-fat
- ❑ yogurt, artificially sweetened raspberry-flavored nonfat
- ❑ yogurt, artificially sweetened vanilla
- ❑ yogurt, plain lowfat

Frozen Foods
- ❑ broccoli

Meat and Poultry
- ❑ Canadian bacon
- ❑ chicken breasts, boneless and skinless
- ❑ chicken, roasted
- ❑ ham, thinly sliced
- ❑ roast beef, boneless and thinly sliced
- ❑ steak, top round
- ❑ veggie ground round

Second Week Meals and Recipes

DAY 1

Breakfast

Low-fat Pancakes

3 large eggs
1 cup plain low-fat yogurt
$1/4$ cup unsweetened applesauce
$1/2$ tsp. vanilla extract
2 tbsp. sugar or Splenda® equivalent

1 tsp. baking soda
$1/4$ tsp. salt
1 cup all-purpose flour
1 cup blueberries
nonstick cooking spray

Separate 1 egg white and yolk into 2 large bowls. Add whites only from remaining 2 eggs into egg-white bowl; save extra yolks in refrigerator for another recipe. Add yogurt, applesauce, vanilla and sugar to egg-yolk bowl and stir with rubber spatula to mix. Stir in baking soda, salt and flour, and blend well. Beat egg whites with an electric mixer until stiff peaks form when the beaters are lifted. Stir $1/3$ of the egg whites into batter until blended, and then gently fold in remaining whites until no white streaks remain. Next, preheat a griddle (or a large skillet) over medium heat until a few drops of water flicked onto the surface skitter around and then disappear. Coat the griddle with cooking spray. Pour $1/4$ cup batter onto griddle, and then gently spread to make a 4-inch pancake. If you are using fruit for this recipe, quickly sprinkle on top (note that you can substitute an equal amount of raspberries, chopped apples or pears for the blueberries). Cook 2 minutes more or until bubbles appear on surface of pancake and the underside is golden brown. Turn the pancake over with broad metal spatula and cook for 2 more minutes (until tops bounce back when touched). Makes 4 servings of 3 pancakes or 6 servings of 2 pancakes.

Nutritional Information: 261 calories; 5g fat (17.8% calories from fat); 11g protein; 42g carbohydrate; 2g dietary fiber; 163mg cholesterol; 547mg sodium.

Lunch

6-oz. baked potato, topped with1 tsp. reduced-calorie margarine, $1/2$ cup cooked chopped spinach, and 1$1/2$ oz. grated reduced-fat cheddar cheese

Serve with 1 cup carrot sticks and 1 cup celery sticks.

Nutritional Information: 344 calories; 5g fat (13.8% calories from fat); 17g protein; 59g carbohydrate; 10g dietary fiber; 9mg cholesterol; 479mg sodium.

Dinner

Oven-Fried Chicken (or Fish)

(4) 4-oz. boneless, skinless chicken breasts (or substitute fish fillets)

$^1/_2$ cup *All-Purpose Breading Mix*
nonstick cooking spray

Preheat oven to 425° F. Place *All-Purpose Breading Mix* (see additional recipes section) in a shallow pan. Spray each breast (or fillet) with cooking spray and coat each side with breading mixture. Arrange in 9″ x 9″ baking dish coated with cooking spray. Bake 15 to 20 minutes. Serve each with 1 cup steamed sugar snap peas and a 3-ounce baked potato topped with 1 teaspoon reduced-fat margarine and reduced-fat sour cream. Serves 4.

Nutritional Information: 349 calories; 5g fat (14.3% calories from fat); 33g protein; 40g carbohydrate; 6g dietary fiber; 70mg cholesterol; 519mg sodium.

DAY 2

Breakfast

$^1/_2$ large (4 oz.) whole-wheat bagel, toasted and topped with 1 tbsp. fat-free cream cheese

Serve with 1 small orange and 1 cup nonfat milk.

Nutritional Information: 286 calories; 2g fat (4.7% calories from fat); 17g protein; 53g carbohydrate; 6g dietary fiber; 6mg cholesterol; 427mg sodium.

Lunch

Egg Salad Muffin with Broccoli Bisque

1 English muffin, toasted
2 cups frozen, chopped broccoli
$^1/_2$ cup low-sodium chicken broth
$^1/_2$ cup nonfat milk
2 hard-boiled egg whites, chopped

1 hard-boiled egg with yolk, chopped
1 tbsp. finely chopped celery
2 tsp. low-fat mayonnaise
salt and pepper to taste

Combine broccoli, chicken broth and milk in food processor and purée until smooth. Combine eggs, celery, mayonnaise, salt and pepper in a small bowl. Mix well and set aside. Transfer broccoli mixture to saucepan and cook over medium heat until hot. While heating the bisque, scoop egg mixture onto a toasted English muffin. Serve with 1 small apple. Serves 1.

Nutritional Information: 493 calories; 12g fat (19.9% calories from fat); 36g protein; 71g carbohydrate; 15g dietary fiber; 218mg cholesterol; 648mg sodium.

Dinner

Chicken and Broccoli Frittata

$1^1/_2$ cups chopped roasted chicken
2 cups chopped broccoli florets
2 tbsp. dry bread crumbs
3 tbsp. all-purpose flour
1 tsp. dried basil
$^1/_4$ tsp. salt
$^1/_8$ tsp. pepper

1 cup nonfat milk
1 tsp. Dijon mustard
(1) 4-oz. carton egg substitute
$^1/_2$ cup shredded, reduced-fat, extra-sharp cheddar cheese, divided
$^1/_2$ tsp. paprika
nonstick cooking spray

Preheat oven to 350° F. Cook broccoli in boiling water for 3 minutes or until tender-crisp. Drain and set aside. Coat a 9″ pie pan with cooking spray, and then sprinkle with breadcrumbs (do not remove the excess crumbs). Set the breadcrumbs aside. In a large bowl, combine flour, basil, salt and pepper, and then add the milk and mustard. Blend well with whisk, and then stir in egg substitute. Add chicken and $^1/_4$ cup cheese, stirring well. Pour the mixture into pie pan and sprinkle with remaining cheese and paprika. Bake for 45 minutes or until set. Let cool on rack for 5 minutes before slicing. Serve each with 1 cup green salad with 2 tablespoons low-fat dressing and a 1-ounce dinner roll. Serves 4.

Nutritional Information: 263 calories; 8g fat (28.8% calories from fat); 28g protein; 18g carbohydrate; 2g dietary fiber; 50mg cholesterol; 503mg sodium.

DAY 3

Breakfast

1 English muffin, toasted and topped with 1 oz. slice Canadian bacon (sautéed) and 1 slice tomato

Serve with 1 small orange.

Nutritional Information: 266 calories; 4g fat (11.7% calories from fat); 13g protein; 48g carbohydrate; 6g dietary fiber; 14mg cholesterol; 675mg sodium.

Lunch

Cheese and Veggie Sandwich

2 slices light whole-wheat bread
1-oz. slice reduced-fat Swiss cheese
$1/_4$ cup roasted red bell pepper strips, drained

$1/_4$ cup alfalfa sprouts
$1/_4$ cup spinach leaves
1 tbsp. low-fat Thousand Island dressing

Combine ingredients to make a sandwich. Serve with one 8-oz. can ready-to-eat tomato soup, 6 saltine crackers, 1 cup broccoli florets, and 1 cup artificially sweetened raspberry-flavored nonfat yogurt topped with $1/_2$ cup raspberries.

Nutritional Information: 500 calories; 9g fat (15.3% calories from fat); 29g protein; 83g carbohydrate; 14g dietary fiber; 14mg cholesterol; 1,439mg sodium.

Dinner

Chili non Carne Vegetarian

(2) 12-oz. pkgs. veggie ground round
(1) 15-oz. can each kidney, black and great Northern beans
(2) 16-oz. cans diced tomatoes
2 large onions, chopped

(2) 8-oz. cans tomato sauce
2 green bell peppers, chopped
$1/_4$ tsp. paprika
2 tbsp. chili powder
2 tsp. ground cumin

Combine all ingredients in a large pot and stir to blend well. Bring to a boil, and then cover and simmer for 1 hour. Serve each with 8 crackers and 1 peach. Makes about 3 quarts or 8-1$1/_2$-cup servings.

Nutritional Information: 670 calories; 10g fat (12.9% calories from fat); 29g protein; 123g carbohydrate; 23g dietary fiber; 0mg cholesterol; 616mg sodium.

DAY 4

Breakfast

1 cup cooked oatmeal, topped with $1/_4$ tsp. reduced-fat margarine, a dash of cinnamon, a dash of nutmeg, and 2 tbsp. raisins.

Serve with 1 cup nonfat milk.

Nutritional Information: 284 calories; 3g fat (10.6% calories from fat); 15g protein; 50g carbohydrate; 5g dietary fiber; 4mg cholesterol; 517mg sodium.

Lunch

Roast Beef Sandwich

2 slices light whole-wheat bread
$1^1/_2$ oz. cooked lean, boneless roast
  beef, thinly sliced
2 slices tomato

2 romaine lettuce leaves
1 tbsp. low-fat Thousand Island
  dressing

Serve with $1/_2$ cup celery sticks, $1/_2$ cup carrot sticks, and 1 cup sugar-free, white-grape-flavored gelatin mixed with 1 cup grapes.

Nutritional Information: 416 calories; 9g fat (21% calories from fat); 25g protein; 50g carbohydrate; 7g dietary fiber; 36mg cholesterol; 1,018mg sodium.

Dinner

Spicy Eggplant Casserole

2 small eggplants, peeled and cut
  into 1-in. cubes
$1^1/_2$ tbsp. chopped onion
$1^1/_2$ tbsp. chopped celery
$1^1/_2$ tbsp. chopped bell pepper
$1/_2$ cup soft bread cubes

(1) 10-oz. can diced tomatoes
  with chilies
salt and cayenne pepper (to taste)
2 oz. 2-percent cheddar cheese,
  shredded
nonstick cooking spray

Preheat oven to 400° F. Salt eggplants and let sit for 20 minutes to draw out bitterness. Rinse and drain. In medium bowl, combine eggplants, onion, celery, bell pepper, canned tomatoes, bread cubes, salt and pepper. Pour into 9″ x 9″ baking dish coated with cooking spray. Top with cheese and bake for 20 to 25 minutes. Serve each with 1 cup green salad with 2 tablespoons low-fat dressing and a 1-ounce breadstick. Serves 4.

Nutritional Information: 275 calories; 7g fat (23.1% calories from fat); 12g protein; 44g carbohydrate; 8g dietary fiber; 5mg cholesterol; 849mg sodium.

DAY 5

Breakfast

Raisin French Toast

$1^1/_2$ slices cinnamon-raisin bread
$1/_4$ cup egg substitute
$1/_4$ tsp. vanilla flavoring

1 tbsp. nonfat milk
nonstick cooking spray

Combine egg substitute, vanilla and milk in a shallow bowl. Add slices of bread, turning until egg mixture is absorbed. Spray a small nonstick skillet or griddle with nonstick cooking spray, and preheat. Cook bread over medium heat 3 to 5 minutes, turning once, until golden brown on both sides. Serve with 1 tablespoon sugar-free syrup, $1/2$ cup grapefruit sections and $1/2$ cup nonfat milk. Serves 1.

Nutritional Information: 358 calories; 8g fat (19.7% calories from fat); 17g protein; 55g carbohydrate; 3g dietary fiber; 4mg cholesterol; 371mg sodium.

....

Lunch

Meatloaf Sandwich

1 meatloaf sandwich, made with 1 English muffin (split), 2-oz. slice *Salsa Meatloaf* (see recipe below), 2 tomato slices and 2 romaine lettuce leaves.

Serve with $1/2$ cup artificially sweetened vanilla-flavored nonfat yogurt and 1 cup mixed berries

Nutritional Information: 536 calories; 19g fat (31.4% calories from fat); 27g protein; 65g carbohydrate; 6g dietary fiber; 94mg cholesterol; 876mg sodium.

Salsa Meat Loaf

1 lb. lean (15 percent fat or less) ground beef	1 tsp. salt
	2 slices bread, finely cubed
1 egg	$1/2$ tsp. dry mustard
2 tbsp. finely chopped green pepper	1 cup prepared salsa
1 c. finely chopped onion	

Preheat oven to 400° F. In large bowl, combine all ingredients and mix well to form a loaf. Place loaf in a foil-lined 5″ x 9″ baking pan. Bake 40 to 45 minutes or until done. Serves 4.

....

Dinner

Roasted Chicken with Butternut Squash

2 tbsp. minced garlic	nonstick cooking spray
1 tsp. salt	12 oz. red potatoes, cut into wedges
$3/4$ tsp. freshly ground black pepper	$1^1/2$ cups cubed peeled butternut
$1/2$ teaspoon dried rubbed sage	squash (about 8 oz.)
1 ($3^1/2$-pound) roasting chicken	2 tbsp. butter, melted

Preheat oven to 400° F. Combine 1$^1/_2$ tablespoons garlic, $^1/_2$ teaspoon salt, $^1/_2$ teaspoon pepper and sage in a small bowl. Remove and discard giblets and neck from chicken. Starting at neck cavity, loosen skin from breast and drumsticks by inserting fingers, gently pushing between skin and meat. Lift wing tips up and over back, and then tuck under chicken. Rub the garlic mixture under loosened skin. Place chicken, breast side up, on rack of a broiler pan coated with nonstick cooking spray. Place rack in a broiler pan. Combine potatoes, squash, butter, $^1/_2$ teaspoon garlic, $^1/_2$ teaspoon salt and $^1/_4$ teaspoon pepper. Arrange vegetable mixture around chicken. Bake at 400° F for 1 hour or until a thermometer inserted into meaty part of thigh registers 165° F. Let stand for 10 minutes. Discard skin. Serves 4.

Nutritional Information: 399 calories; 12g fat (34% calories from fat); 43.8g protein; 25.9g carbohydrate; 3.4g dietary fiber; 147mg cholesterol; 791mg sodium.

DAY 6

Breakfast

Quick Breakfast Tostada

$^1/_4$ cup 1-percent low-fat milk
$^1/_8$ tsp. freshly ground black pepper
4 large egg whites
2 large eggs
4 (6-inch) corn tortillas
$^1/_2$ cup (2 oz.) shredded reduced-fat sharp cheddar cheese

1 cup canned black beans, rinsed and drained
$^1/_4$ cup chopped green onions
$^1/_2$ cup bottled salsa
$^1/_4$ cup fat-free sour cream
$^1/_4$ tsp. salt

Combine low-fat milk, salt, pepper, egg whites and eggs in a large microwave-safe dish, stirring with a whisk. Microwave at high for 3 minutes; stir and microwave an additional 1 minute (or until done). Arrange 1 tortilla each on 4 microwave-safe plates, and then divide egg mixture evenly among the corn tortillas. Layer each serving with 2 tablespoons cheese, $^1/_4$ cup beans and 1 tablespoon green onions. Microwave each tostada at high for 30 seconds. Top each tostada with 2 tablespoons salsa and 1 tablespoon sour cream. Serve immediately. Serves 4.

Nutritional Information: 201 calories; 6.5g fat (29% calories from fat); 15.9g protein; 23g carbohydrate; 4.4g dietary fiber; 120mg cholesterol; 633mg sodium.

Lunch

1 cup 90-calorie vegetable soup
20 oyster crackers
(1) 1-oz. slice Italian or French
bread, topped with 1 tsp. reduced-
fat margarine
1 cup strawberries

1 tossed salad, made with
2 cups mixed dark green lettuce
$1/_2$ cup roasted red bell pepper
strips (chilled)
$1/_2$ cup sliced celery
2 oz. reduced-fat cheddar cheese
2 tbsp. low-fat Italian dressing

Nutritional Information: 485 calories; 15g fat (27.0% calories from fat); 25g protein; 66g carbohydrate; 11g dietary fiber; 14mg cholesterol; 1,827mg sodium.

Dinner

Ham and Dijon Mustard Sandwich

1 tbsp. whole-grain Dijon mustard
1 tbsp. fat-free mayonnaise
8 (1-oz) slices Italian bread
6 oz. thinly sliced ham
1 cup (4 oz.) shredded Gruyère cheese

$1/_4$ tsp. freshly ground black pepper
$1/_2$ cup egg substitute
$1/_4$ cup fat-free milk
nonstick cooking spray

Combine mustard and mayonnaise in a small bowl. Spread $3/_4$ teaspoon mustard mixture over each of 4 bread slices, and then layer each slice with $1^1/_2$ ounces ham and $1/_4$ cup cheese. Sprinkle evenly with pepper. Spread $3/_4$ teaspoon mayonnaise mixture over each remaining bread slice, and then place, mustard side down, on top of sandwiches. Combine egg substitute and fat-free milk in a shallow dish. Dip both sides of each sandwich into the egg mixture. Coat a large nonstick griddle or skillet with nonstick cooking spray and heat over medium heat. Add sandwiches to pan. Cook for 3 minutes on each side or until lightly browned and cheese melts.

Nutritional Information: 350 calories; 11.7g fat (30% calories from fat); 25g protein; 34.6g carbohydrate; 1.7g dietary fiber; 51mg cholesterol; 935mg sodium.

DAY 7

Breakfast

Raspberry Walnut Muffins

$2/_3$ cup (5 oz.) reduced-fat cream
cheese, softened

$1/_3$ cup butter, softened
$1^1/_2$ cups sugar

1¹/₂ tsp. vanilla extract
2 large egg whites
1 large egg
2 cups all-purpose flour
1 tsp. baking powder

¹/₄ tsp. baking soda
¹/₂ tsp. salt
¹/₂ cup low-fat buttermilk
2 cups fresh or frozen raspberries
¹/₄ cup finely chopped walnuts

Preheat oven to 350° F. Combine cream cheese and butter in a large bowl, and then beat with a mixer at high speed until well blended. Add sugar, and beat until fluffy. Add vanilla, egg whites and egg; beat well. Lightly spoon flour into dry measuring cups and level with a knife. Combine flour, baking powder, baking soda and salt. With mixer on low speed, add the flour mixture and buttermilk to cream cheese mixture, beginning and ending with flour mixture. Gently fold in raspberries and walnuts. Place 24 foil cup liners in muffin cups and spoon batter evenly into liners. Bake at 350° F for 25 minutes or until a wooden pick inserted in center comes out clean. Remove from pans, and then cool on a wire rack. Serves 12.

Nutritional Information: 142 calories; 4.7 g fat (32% calories from fat); 2.7g protein; 22g carbohydrate; 1g dietary fiber; 19mg cholesterol; 1,138mg sodium.

....

Lunch

BBQ Chicken Salad

12 oz. boneless, skinless chicken
   breasts
2 tsp. mild or hot chili powder
2 tsp. onion powder
1 tsp. garlic powder
1 tsp. paprika
8 cups torn romaine lettuce leaves

2 medium tomatoes, each sliced into
   8 wedges
1 cup cooked corn
2 thin red-onion slices, separated
   into rings
2 tbsp. low-fat Ranch dressing

Preheat oven to 350° F. In a small bowl, combine chili powder, onion powder, garlic powder and paprika. Rub mixture evenly over both sides of chicken breasts. Place chicken onto large sheet of foil and wrap tightly, crimping edges to seal. Place foil packet onto baking sheet and bake for 8 to 10 minutes. Carefully open packet and bake 6 to 8 minutes more, or until chicken is cooked through and juices run clear when pierced with fork. Set aside to cool. While chicken is cooling, line a large bowl with lettuce and then top with tomatoes, corn and onion slices. Shred cooled chicken with fork and add to lettuce mixture. Drizzle evenly with dressing. Serve with 1 cup broccoli florets, a 1-ounce whole-wheat roll with 1 teaspoon reduced-calorie margarine, and 1 medium peach. Serves 4.

Nutritional Information: 423 calories; 9g fat (16.7% calories from fat); 35g protein; 61g carbohydrate; 18g dietary fiber; 53mg cholesterol; 389mg sodium.

....

Dinner

Pepper Steak

1 tsp. olive oil
2 cups sliced onion
2 cups green bell pepper strips
2 tsp. bottled minced garlic
1 cup sliced mushrooms
$^3/_4$ lb. top round steak, trimmed and
   cut into thin strips

$^1/_4$ tsp. salt
$^1/_8$ tsp. black pepper
2 tsp. Worcestershire sauce
4 slices reduced-fat provolone cheese,
   cut in half
4 ($2^1/_2$-ounce) hoagie rolls with
   sesame seeds

Heat oil in a large nonstick skillet over medium-high heat. Add onion, bell pepper and garlic to pan and sauté for 3 minutes. Add mushrooms to pan and sauté for 4 minutes. Sprinkle beef with salt and black pepper. Add beef to pan and sauté for 3 minutes or until browned, stirring occasionally. Stir in Worcestershire sauce and cook for 1 minute. Place 1 cheese slice half on bottom half of each roll and top each serving with $^1/_4$ of the beef mixture. Top with remaining cheese slice halves and tops of rolls. Serves 4.

Nutritional Information: 384 calories; 9.8g fat (23% calories from fat); 32.9g protein; 44.9g carbohydrate; 4g dietary fiber; 43mg cholesterol; 580mg sodium.

HEALTHY SNACK CHOICES
(**Note:** Add the ingredients for each of these items to the grocery lists.)

- 30 small pretzel sticks
- $^3/_4$ cup fiber-rich or grain cereal
- 2 gingersnaps
- 1 low-fat, sugar-free fruit yogurt cup
- cucumber slices lightly salted or with nonfat Italian dressing
- 1 cup frozen berries (grapes are great frozen!)
- 4 cups air-popped/light popcorn
- 1 mini-bagel (1 oz.) with 2 oz. fat-free cream cheese
- 1 banana-chocolate whip (combine 1 cup fat-free milk, 1 small banana, a squeeze of chocolate syrup and a handful of ice cubes in a blender)
- 15 baby carrots and 2 tablespoons fat-free Ranch dressing

ADDITIONAL RECIPES
(**Note:** Add the ingredients for each of these items to the grocery lists.)

Power Breakfast Smoothie

$3/_4$ cup nonfat plain yogurt
1 cup orange juice
$3/_4$ cup peeled, diced apple
1 medium banana, frozen

1 tsp. vanilla extract
3 tbsp. smooth peanut butter
2 tbsp. wheat germ

Combine all ingredients in a blender and purée until smooth. Serves 4.

Nutritional Information: 179 calories; 7g fat (33.2% calories from fat); 7g protein; 24g carbohydrate; 3g dietary fiber; 1mg cholesterol; 90mg sodium.

All-Purpose Breading Mix

1 cup packaged cornflake crumbs
$1/_4$ tsp. granulated garlic
1 tsp. paprika
$1/_4$ tsp. onion powder

1 tsp. instant chicken bouillon
$1/_8$ tsp. black pepper
$1/_2$ tsp. poultry seasoning

Combine all ingredients and mix well. Store in an airtight container and mix well before using. Makes about 1 cup. Plan on using 2 tablespoons for each chicken breast (you can substitute fish fillet for chicken). Serves 8.

Nutritional Information: 13 calories; 1g fat (19.3% calories from fat); 1g protein; 3g carbohydrate; 1g dietary fiber; 0mg cholesterol; 2mg sodium.

Corn Salsa

$1^1/_2$ cups corn kernels
$1/_4$ cup chopped red onion
$1/_4$ cup chopped red bell pepper
$1/_4$ cup chopped fresh cilantro

$1^1/_2$ tbsp. fresh lime juice
1 to 2 tsp. seeded chopped jalapeño peppers
salt and pepper (to taste)

Combine all ingredients in large bowl; refrigerate until needed. Makes 4 servings. (Note: the salsa may be made the day before using—cover and refrigerate until needed.)

Nutritional Information: 62 calories; 1g fat (6.4% calories from fat); 2g protein; 15g carbohydrate; 2g dietary fiber; 0mg cholesterol; 3mg sodium.

Member Survey

Please answer the following questions to help your leader plan your First Place 4 Health meetings so that your needs might be met in this session. Give this form to your leader at the first group meeting.

Name _____ Birth date _____

Please list those who live in your household.

Name	Relationship	Age

What church do you attend? _____

Are you interested in receiving more information about our church?

          Yes   No

Occupation _____

What talent or area of expertise would you be willing to share with our class?

_____

Why did you join First Place 4 Health?

_____

With notice, would you be willing to lead a Bible study discussion one week?

          Yes   No

Are you comfortable praying out loud? _____

If the assistant leader were absent, would you be willing to assist in weighing in members and possibly evaluating the Live It Trackers?

          Yes   No

Any other comments:

_____

_____

Personal Weight and Measurement Record

Week	Weight	+ or -	Goal this Session	Pounds to goal
1				
2				
3				
4				
5				
6				
7				
8				
9				
10				
11				
12				

Beginning Measurements

Waist _____ Hips _____ Thighs _____ Chest _____

Ending Measurements

Waist _____ Hips _____ Thighs _____ Chest _____

Rec'd step 3 pg 182

First Place 4 Health
Prayer Partner

THE POWER
OF HOPE
Week
3

Hope deferred makes the heart sick, but a longing fulfilled is a tree of life.

Proverbs 13:12

Date: 7·3·12

Name: Bonnie

Home Phone: 508 209 4940

Work Phone: (

Email: VCC @ Vineyard crossroads. org

Personal Prayer Concerns:

Salvation for Son Joseph, Daughter
Bethany, grandson - Jacob, Braedan
grandaughter Zoey,

That I would stay focused on the
love of God and His love for me

This form is for prayer requests that are personal to you and your journey in First Place 4 Health. Please complete this form and have it ready to turn in when you arrive at your group meeting.

First Place 4 Health
Prayer Partner

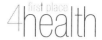

THE POWER
OF HOPE
Week
4

Be joyful in hope, patient in affliction, faithful in prayer.
ROMANS 12:12

Date: _____

Name: _____

Home Phone: (_____) _____

Work Phone: (_____) _____

Email: _____

Personal Prayer Concerns:

_____

_____

_____

_____

_____

_____

_____

This form is for prayer requests that are personal to you and your journey in First Place 4 Health. Please complete this form and have it ready to turn in when you arrive at your group meeting.

First Place 4 Health
Prayer Partner

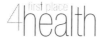

THE POWER
OF HOPE
Week
5

SCRIPTURE VERSE TO MEMORIZE FOR WEEK SIX:
*Now faith is being sure of what we hope for
and certain of what we do not see.*
HEBREWS 11:1

Date: _____

Name: _____

Home Phone: (____) _____

Work Phone: (____) _____

Email: _____

Personal Prayer Concerns:

_____

_____

_____

_____

_____

_____

_____

This form is for prayer requests that are personal to you and your journey in First Place 4 Health. Please complete this form and have it ready to turn in when you arrive at your group meeting.

First Place 4 Health
Prayer Partner

THE POWER
OF HOPE
Week
6

Date: _____

Name: _____

Home Phone: (_____) _____

Work Phone: (_____) _____

Email: _____

Personal Prayer Concerns:

_____

_____

_____

_____

_____

_____

_____

First Place 4 Health
Prayer Partner

THE POWER
OF HOPE
Week
7

SCRIPTURE VERSE TO MEMORIZE FOR WEEK EIGHT:

Why do you call me "Lord, Lord," and do not do what I say?

LUKE 6:46

Date: _____

Name: _____

Home Phone: _____

Work Phone: _____

Email: _____

Personal Prayer Concerns:

_____

_____

_____

_____

_____

_____

_____

This form is for prayer requests that are personal to you and your journey in First Place 4 Health. Please complete this form and have it ready to turn in when you arrive at your group meeting.

First Place 4 Health
Prayer Partner

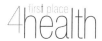

THE POWER
OF HOPE
Week
9

SCRIPTURE VERSE TO MEMORIZE FOR WEEK TEN:

And hope does not disappoint us, because God has poured out his love
into our hearts by the Holy Spirit, whom he has given us.
ROMANS 5:5

Date: _____

Name: _____

Home Phone: _____

Work Phone: _____

Email: _____

Personal Prayer Concerns:

_____

_____

_____

_____

_____

_____

_____

This form is for prayer requests that are personal to you and your journey in First Place 4 Health. Please complete this form and have it ready to turn in when you arrive at your group meeting.

First Place 4 Health
Prayer Partner

4 first place
health

THE POWER
OF HOPE
Week
10

SCRIPTURE VERSE TO MEMORIZE FOR WEEK ELEVEN:
But as for me, I will always have hope; I will praise you more and more.
PSALM 71:14

Date: _____

Name: _____

Home Phone: (_____) _____

Work Phone: (_____) _____

Email: _____

Personal Prayer Concerns:

_____

_____

_____

_____

_____

_____

_____

This form is for prayer requests that are personal to you and your journey in First Place 4 Health. Please complete this form and have it ready to turn in when you arrive at your group meeting.

First Place 4 Health
Prayer Partner

Date: _____

Name: _____

Home Phone: (_____) _____

Work Phone: (_____) _____

Email: _____

Personal Prayer Concerns:

_____

_____

_____

_____

_____

_____

_____

This form is for prayer requests that are personal to you and your journey in First Place 4 Health. Please complete this form and have it ready to turn in when you arrive at your group meeting.

Live It Tracker

Name: _____ Loss/gain: _____ lbs.

Date: _____ Week #: ____ Calorie Range: _____ My food goal for next week: _____

Activity Level: None, < 30 min/day, 30-60 min/day, 60+ min/day My activity goal for next week: _____

Group	Daily Calories							
	1300-1400	1500-1600	1700-1800	1900-2000	2100-2200	2300-2400	2500-2600	2700-2800
Fruits	1.5-2 c.	1.5-2 c.	1.5-2 c.	2-2.5 c.	2-2.5 c.	2.5-3.5 c.	3.5-4.5 c.	3.5-4.5 c.
Vegetables	1.5-2 c.	2-2.5 c.	2.5-3 c.	2.5-3 c.	3-3.5 c.	3.5-4.5 c.	4.5-5 c.	4.5-5 c.
Grains	5 oz-eq.	5-6 oz-eq.	6-7 oz-eq.	6-7 oz-eq.	7-8 oz-eq.	8-9 oz-eq.	9-10 oz-eq.	10-11 oz-eq.
Meat & Beans	4 oz-eq.	5 oz-eq.	5-5.5 oz-eq.	5.5-6.5 oz-eq.	6.5-7 oz-eq.	7-7.5 oz-eq.	7-7.5 oz-eq.	7.5-8 oz-eq.
Milk	2-3 c.	3 c.	3 c.	3 c.	3 c.	3 c.	3 c.	3 c.
Healthy Oils	4 tsp.	5 tsp.	5 tsp.	6 tsp.	6 tsp.	7 tsp.	8 tsp.	8 tsp.

Day/Date:

Breakfast: _____ Lunch: _____

Dinner: _____ Snack: _____

Group	Fruits	Vegetables	Grains	Meat & Beans	Milk	Oils
Goal Amount						
Estimate Your Total						
Increase ⇧ or Decrease? ⇩						

Physical Activity: _____ Spiritual Activity: _____

Steps/Miles/Minutes: _____

Day/Date:

Breakfast: _____ Lunch: _____

Dinner: _____ Snack: _____

Group	Fruits	Vegetables	Grains	Meat & Beans	Milk	Oils
Goal Amount						
Estimate Your Total						
Increase ⇧ or Decrease? ⇩						

Physical Activity: _____ Spiritual Activity: _____

Steps/Miles/Minutes: _____

Day/Date:

Breakfast: _____ Lunch: _____

Dinner: _____ Snack: _____

Group	Fruits	Vegetables	Grains	Meat & Beans	Milk	Oils
Goal Amount						
Estimate Your Total						
Increase ⇧ or Decrease? ⇩						

Physical Activity: _____ Spiritual Activity: _____

Steps/Miles/Minutes: _____

Day/Date: ___

Breakfast: _____ Lunch: _____

Dinner: _____ Snack: _____

Group	Fruits	Vegetables	Grains	Meat & Beans	Milk	Oils
Goal Amount						
Estimate Your Total						
Increase ⬆ or Decrease? ⬇						

Physical Activity: _____ Spiritual Activity: _____

Steps/Miles/Minutes: _____ _____

Day/Date: ___

Breakfast: _____ Lunch: _____

Dinner: _____ Snack: _____

Group	Fruits	Vegetables	Grains	Meat & Beans	Milk	Oils
Goal Amount						
Estimate Your Total						
Increase ⬆ or Decrease? ⬇						

Physical Activity: _____ Spiritual Activity: _____

Steps/Miles/Minutes: _____ _____

Day/Date: ___

Breakfast: _____ Lunch: _____

Dinner: _____ Snack: _____

Group	Fruits	Vegetables	Grains	Meat & Beans	Milk	Oils
Goal Amount						
Estimate Your Total						
Increase ⬆ or Decrease? ⬇						

Physical Activity: _____ Spiritual Activity: _____

Steps/Miles/Minutes: _____ _____

Day/Date: ___

Breakfast: _____ Lunch: _____

Dinner: _____ Snack: _____

Group	Fruits	Vegetables	Grains	Meat & Beans	Milk	Oils
Goal Amount						
Estimate Your Total						
Increase ⬆ or Decrease? ⬇						

Physical Activity: _____ Spiritual Activity: _____

Steps/Miles/Minutes: _____ _____

Live It Tracker

Name: _____ Loss/gain: _____ lbs.

Date: _____ Week #: _____ Calorie Range: _____ My food goal for next week: _____

Activity Level: None, < 30 min/day, 30-60 min/day, 60+ min/day My activity goal for next week: _____

Group	Daily Calories							
	1300-1400	1500-1600	1700-1800	1900-2000	2100-2200	2300-2400	2500-2600	2700-2800
Fruits	1.5-2 c.	1.5-2 c.	1.5-2 c.	2-2.5 c.	2-2.5 c.	2.5-3.5 c.	3.5-4.5 c.	3.5-4.5 c.
Vegetables	1.5-2 c.	2-2.5 c.	2.5-3 c.	2.5-3 c.	3-3.5 c.	3.5-4.5 c.	4.5-5 c.	4.5-5 c.
Grains	5 oz-eq.	5-6 oz-eq.	6-7 oz-eq.	6-7 oz-eq.	7-8 oz-eq.	8-9 oz-eq.	9-10 oz-eq.	10-11 oz-eq.
Meat & Beans	4 oz-eq.	5 oz-eq.	5-5.5 oz-eq.	5.5-6.5 oz-eq.	6.5-7 oz-eq.	7-7.5 oz-eq.	7-7.5 oz-eq.	7.5-8 oz-eq.
Milk	2-3 c.	3 c.	3 c.	3 c.	3 c.	3 c.	3 c.	3 c.
Healthy Oils	4 tsp.	5 tsp.	5 tsp.	6 tsp.	6 tsp.	7 tsp.	8 tsp.	8 tsp.

Day/Date: _____

Breakfast: _____ Lunch: _____

Dinner: _____ Snack: _____

Group	Fruits	Vegetables	Grains	Meat & Beans	Milk	Oils
Goal Amount						
Estimate Your Total						
Increase ⇧ or Decrease? ⇩						

Physical Activity: _____ Spiritual Activity: _____

Steps/Miles/Minutes: _____ _____

Day/Date: _____

Breakfast: _____ Lunch: _____

Dinner: _____ Snack: _____

Group	Fruits	Vegetables	Grains	Meat & Beans	Milk	Oils
Goal Amount						
Estimate Your Total						
Increase ⇧ or Decrease? ⇩						

Physical Activity: _____ Spiritual Activity: _____

Steps/Miles/Minutes: _____ _____

Day/Date: _____

Breakfast: _____ Lunch: _____

Dinner: _____ Snack: _____

Group	Fruits	Vegetables	Grains	Meat & Beans	Milk	Oils
Goal Amount						
Estimate Your Total						
Increase ⇧ or Decrease? ⇩						

Physical Activity: _____ Spiritual Activity: _____

Steps/Miles/Minutes: _____

Day/Date:

Breakfast: _____   Lunch: _____

Dinner: _____   Snack: _____

Group	Fruits	Vegetables	Grains	Meat & Beans	Milk	Oils
Goal Amount						
Estimate Your Total						
Increase ⇧ or Decrease? ⇩						

Physical Activity: _____   Spiritual Activity: _____

Steps/Miles/Minutes: _____   _____

Day/Date:

Breakfast: _____   Lunch: _____

Dinner: _____   Snack: _____

Group	Fruits	Vegetables	Grains	Meat & Beans	Milk	Oils
Goal Amount						
Estimate Your Total						
Increase ⇧ or Decrease? ⇩						

Physical Activity: _____   Spiritual Activity: _____

Steps/Miles/Minutes: _____   _____

Day/Date:

Breakfast: _____   Lunch: _____

Dinner: _____   Snack: _____

Group	Fruits	Vegetables	Grains	Meat & Beans	Milk	Oils
Goal Amount						
Estimate Your Total						
Increase ⇧ or Decrease? ⇩						

Physical Activity: _____   Spiritual Activity: _____

Steps/Miles/Minutes: _____   _____

Day/Date:

Breakfast: _____   Lunch: _____

Dinner: _____   Snack: _____

Group	Fruits	Vegetables	Grains	Meat & Beans	Milk	Oils
Goal Amount						
Estimate Your Total						
Increase ⇧ or Decrease? ⇩						

Physical Activity: _____   Spiritual Activity: _____

Steps/Miles/Minutes: _____   _____

Live It Tracker

Name: _____ Loss/gain: _____ lbs.

Date: _____ Week #: ____ Calorie Range: _____ My food goal for next week: _____

Activity Level: None, < 30 min/day, 30-60 min/day, 60+ min/day My activity goal for next week: _____

Group	Daily Calories							
	1300-1400	1500-1600	1700-1800	1900-2000	2100-2200	2300-2400	2500-2600	2700-2800
Fruits	1.5-2 c.	1.5-2 c.	1.5-2 c.	2-2.5 c.	2-2.5 c.	2.5-3.5 c.	3.5-4.5 c.	3.5-4.5 c.
Vegetables	1.5-2 c.	2-2.5 c.	2.5-3 c.	2.5-3 c.	3-3.5 c.	3.5-4.5 c.	4.5-5 c.	4.5-5 c.
Grains	5 oz-eq.	5-6 oz-eq.	6-7 oz-eq.	6-7 oz-eq.	7-8 oz-eq.	8-9 oz-eq.	9-10 oz-eq.	10-11 oz-eq.
Meat & Beans	4 oz-eq.	5 oz-eq.	5-5.5 oz-eq.	5.5-6.5 oz-eq.	6.5-7 oz-eq.	7-7.5 oz-eq.	7-7.5 oz-eq.	7.5-8 oz-eq.
Milk	2-3 c.	3 c.	3 c.	3 c.	3 c.	3 c.	3 c.	3 c.
Healthy Oils	4 tsp.	5 tsp.	5 tsp.	6 tsp.	6 tsp.	7 tsp.	8 tsp.	8 tsp.

Day/Date: _____

Breakfast: _____ Lunch: _____

Dinner: _____ Snack: _____

Group	Fruits	Vegetables	Grains	Meat & Beans	Milk	Oils
Goal Amount						
Estimate Your Total						
Increase ⇧ or Decrease? ⇩						

Physical Activity: _____ Spiritual Activity: _____

Steps/Miles/Minutes: _____

Day/Date: _____

Breakfast: _____ Lunch: _____

Dinner: _____ Snack: _____

Group	Fruits	Vegetables	Grains	Meat & Beans	Milk	Oils
Goal Amount						
Estimate Your Total						
Increase ⇧ or Decrease? ⇩						

Physical Activity: _____ Spiritual Activity: _____

Steps/Miles/Minutes: _____

Day/Date: _____

Breakfast: _____ Lunch: _____

Dinner: _____ Snack: _____

Group	Fruits	Vegetables	Grains	Meat & Beans	Milk	Oils
Goal Amount						
Estimate Your Total						
Increase ⇧ or Decrease? ⇩						

Physical Activity: _____ Spiritual Activity: _____

Steps/Miles/Minutes: _____

Day/Date: _____

Breakfast: _____   Lunch: _____

Dinner: _____   Snack: _____

Group	Fruits	Vegetables	Grains	Meat & Beans	Milk	Oils
Goal Amount						
Estimate Your Total						
Increase ⇧ or Decrease? ⇩						

Physical Activity: _____   Spiritual Activity: _____

Steps/Miles/Minutes: _____   _____

Day/Date: _____

Breakfast: _____   Lunch: _____

Dinner: _____   Snack: _____

Group	Fruits	Vegetables	Grains	Meat & Beans	Milk	Oils
Goal Amount						
Estimate Your Total						
Increase ⇧ or Decrease? ⇩						

Physical Activity: _____   Spiritual Activity: _____

Steps/Miles/Minutes: _____   _____

Day/Date: _____

Breakfast: _____   Lunch: _____

Dinner: _____   Snack: _____

Group	Fruits	Vegetables	Grains	Meat & Beans	Milk	Oils
Goal Amount						
Estimate Your Total						
Increase ⇧ or Decrease? ⇩						

Physical Activity: _____   Spiritual Activity: _____

Steps/Miles/Minutes: _____   _____

Day/Date: _____

Breakfast: _____   Lunch: _____

Dinner: _____   Snack: _____

Group	Fruits	Vegetables	Grains	Meat & Beans	Milk	Oils
Goal Amount						
Estimate Your Total						
Increase ⇧ or Decrease? ⇩						

Physical Activity: _____   Spiritual Activity: _____

Steps/Miles/Minutes: _____   _____

Live It Tracker

Name: _____ Loss/gain: _____ lbs.

Date: _____ Week #: ____ Calorie Range: _____ My food goal for next week: _____

Activity Level: None, < 30 min/day, 30-60 min/day, 60+ min/day My activity goal for next week: _____

Group	Daily Calories							
	1300-1400	1500-1600	1700-1800	1900-2000	2100-2200	2300-2400	2500-2600	2700-2800
Fruits	1.5-2 c.	1.5-2 c.	1.5-2 c.	2-2.5 c.	2-2.5 c.	2.5-3.5 c.	3.5-4.5 c.	3.5-4.5 c.
Vegetables	1.5-2 c.	2-2.5 c.	2.5-3 c.	2.5-3 c.	3-3.5 c.	3.5-4.5 c.	4.5-5 c.	4.5-5 c.
Grains	5 oz-eq.	5-6 oz-eq.	6-7 oz-eq.	6-7 oz-eq.	7-8 oz-eq.	8-9 oz-eq.	9-10 oz-eq.	10-11 oz-eq.
Meat & Beans	4 oz-eq.	5 oz-eq.	5-5.5 oz-eq.	5.5-6.5 oz-eq.	6.5-7 oz-eq.	7-7.5 oz-eq.	7-7.5 oz-eq.	7.5-8 oz-eq.
Milk	2-3 c.	3 c.	3 c.	3 c.	3 c.	3 c.	3 c.	3 c.
Healthy Oils	4 tsp.	5 tsp.	5 tsp.	6 tsp.	6 tsp.	7 tsp.	8 tsp.	8 tsp.

Day/Date: _____

Breakfast: _____ Lunch: _____

Dinner: _____ Snack: _____

Group	Fruits	Vegetables	Grains	Meat & Beans	Milk	Oils
Goal Amount						
Estimate Your Total						
Increase ⇧ or Decrease? ⇩						

Physical Activity: _____ Spiritual Activity: _____

Steps/Miles/Minutes: _____

Day/Date: _____

Breakfast: _____ Lunch: _____

Dinner: _____ Snack: _____

Group	Fruits	Vegetables	Grains	Meat & Beans	Milk	Oils
Goal Amount						
Estimate Your Total						
Increase ⇧ or Decrease? ⇩						

Physical Activity: _____ Spiritual Activity: _____

Steps/Miles/Minutes: _____

Day/Date: _____

Breakfast: _____ Lunch: _____

Dinner: _____ Snack: _____

Group	Fruits	Vegetables	Grains	Meat & Beans	Milk	Oils
Goal Amount						
Estimate Your Total						
Increase ⇧ or Decrease? ⇩						

Physical Activity: _____ Spiritual Activity: _____

Steps/Miles/Minutes: _____

Day/Date: _____

Breakfast: _____   Lunch: _____

Dinner: _____   Snack: _____

Group	Fruits	Vegetables	Grains	Meat & Beans	Milk	Oils
Goal Amount						
Estimate Your Total						
Increase ⬆ or Decrease? ⬇						

Physical Activity: _____   Spiritual Activity: _____

Steps/Miles/Minutes: _____   _____

Day/Date: _____

Breakfast: _____   Lunch: _____

Dinner: _____   Snack: _____

Group	Fruits	Vegetables	Grains	Meat & Beans	Milk	Oils
Goal Amount						
Estimate Your Total						
Increase ⬆ or Decrease? ⬇						

Physical Activity: _____   Spiritual Activity: _____

Steps/Miles/Minutes: _____   _____

Day/Date: _____

Breakfast: _____   Lunch: _____

Dinner: _____   Snack: _____

Group	Fruits	Vegetables	Grains	Meat & Beans	Milk	Oils
Goal Amount						
Estimate Your Total						
Increase ⬆ or Decrease? ⬇						

Physical Activity: _____   Spiritual Activity: _____

Steps/Miles/Minutes: _____   _____

Day/Date: _____

Breakfast: _____   Lunch: _____

Dinner: _____   Snack: _____

Group	Fruits	Vegetables	Grains	Meat & Beans	Milk	Oils
Goal Amount						
Estimate Your Total						
Increase ⬆ or Decrease? ⬇						

Physical Activity: _____   Spiritual Activity: _____

Steps/Miles/Minutes: _____   _____

Live It Tracker

Name: _____ Loss/gain: _____ lbs.

Date: _____ Week #: _____ Calorie Range: _____ My food goal for next week: _____

Activity Level: None, < 30 min/day, 30-60 min/day, 60+ min/day My activity goal for next week: _____

Group	Daily Calories							
	1300-1400	1500-1600	1700-1800	1900-2000	2100-2200	2300-2400	2500-2600	2700-2800
Fruits	1.5-2 c.	1.5-2 c.	1.5-2 c.	2-2.5 c.	2-2.5 c.	2.5-3.5 c.	3.5-4.5 c.	3.5-4.5 c.
Vegetables	1.5-2 c.	2-2.5 c.	2.5-3 c.	2.5-3 c.	3-3.5 c.	3.5-4.5 c.	4.5-5 c.	4.5-5 c.
Grains	5 oz-eq.	5-6 oz-eq.	6-7 oz-eq.	6-7 oz-eq.	7-8 oz-eq.	8-9 oz-eq.	9-10 oz-eq.	10-11 oz-eq.
Meat & Beans	4 oz-eq.	5 oz-eq.	5-5.5 oz-eq.	5.5-6.5 oz-eq.	6.5-7 oz-eq.	7-7.5 oz-eq.	7-7.5 oz-eq.	7.5-8 oz-eq.
Milk	2-3 c.	3 c.	3 c.	3 c.	3 c.	3 c.	3 c.	3 c.
Healthy Oils	4 tsp.	5 tsp.	5 tsp.	6 tsp.	6 tsp.	7 tsp.	8 tsp.	8 tsp.

Day/Date: _____

Breakfast: _____ Lunch: _____

Dinner: _____ Snack: _____

Group	Fruits	Vegetables	Grains	Meat & Beans	Milk	Oils
Goal Amount						
Estimate Your Total						
Increase ⇧ or Decrease? ⇩						

Physical Activity: _____ Spiritual Activity: _____

Steps/Miles/Minutes: _____

Day/Date: _____

Breakfast: _____ Lunch: _____

Dinner: _____ Snack: _____

Group	Fruits	Vegetables	Grains	Meat & Beans	Milk	Oils
Goal Amount						
Estimate Your Total						
Increase ⇧ or Decrease? ⇩						

Physical Activity: _____ Spiritual Activity: _____

Steps/Miles/Minutes: _____

Day/Date: _____

Breakfast: _____ Lunch: _____

Dinner: _____ Snack: _____

Group	Fruits	Vegetables	Grains	Meat & Beans	Milk	Oils
Goal Amount						
Estimate Your Total						
Increase ⇧ or Decrease? ⇩						

Physical Activity: _____ Spiritual Activity: _____

Steps/Miles/Minutes: _____

Day/Date:

Breakfast: _____ Lunch: _____

Dinner: _____ Snack: _____

Group	Fruits	Vegetables	Grains	Meat & Beans	Milk	Oils
Goal Amount						
Estimate Your Total						
Increase ⇧ or Decrease? ⇩						

Physical Activity: _____ Spiritual Activity: _____

Steps/Miles/Minutes: _____ _____

Day/Date:

Breakfast: _____ Lunch: _____

Dinner: _____ Snack: _____

Group	Fruits	Vegetables	Grains	Meat & Beans	Milk	Oils
Goal Amount						
Estimate Your Total						
Increase ⇧ or Decrease? ⇩						

Physical Activity: _____ Spiritual Activity: _____

Steps/Miles/Minutes: _____ _____

Day/Date:

Breakfast: _____ Lunch: _____

Dinner: _____ Snack: _____

Group	Fruits	Vegetables	Grains	Meat & Beans	Milk	Oils
Goal Amount						
Estimate Your Total						
Increase ⇧ or Decrease? ⇩						

Physical Activity: _____ Spiritual Activity: _____

Steps/Miles/Minutes: _____ _____

Day/Date:

Breakfast: _____ Lunch: _____

Dinner: _____ Snack: _____

Group	Fruits	Vegetables	Grains	Meat & Beans	Milk	Oils
Goal Amount						
Estimate Your Total						
Increase ⇧ or Decrease? ⇩						

Physical Activity: _____ Spiritual Activity: _____

Steps/Miles/Minutes: _____

Live It Tracker

Name: _____ Loss/gain: _____ lbs.

Date: _____ Week #: _____ Calorie Range: _____ My food goal for next week: _____

Activity Level: None, < 30 min/day, 30-60 min/day, 60+ min/day My activity goal for next week: _____

Group	Daily Calories							
	1300-1400	1500-1600	1700-1800	1900-2000	2100-2200	2300-2400	2500-2600	2700-2800
Fruits	1.5-2 c.	1.5-2 c.	1.5-2 c.	2-2.5 c.	2-2.5 c.	2.5-3.5 c.	3.5-4.5 c.	3.5-4.5 c.
Vegetables	1.5-2 c.	2-2.5 c.	2.5-3 c.	2.5-3 c.	3-3.5 c.	3.5-4.5 c.	4.5-5 c.	4.5-5 c.
Grains	5 oz-eq.	5-6 oz-eq.	6-7 oz-eq.	6-7 oz-eq.	7-8 oz-eq.	8-9 oz-eq.	9-10 oz-eq.	10-11 oz-eq.
Meat & Beans	4 oz-eq.	5 oz-eq.	5-5.5 oz-eq.	5.5-6.5 oz-eq.	6.5-7 oz-eq.	7-7.5 oz-eq.	7-7.5 oz-eq.	7.5-8 oz-eq.
Milk	2-3 c.	3 c.	3 c.	3 c.	3 c.	3 c.	3 c.	3 c.
Healthy Oils	4 tsp.	5 tsp.	5 tsp.	6 tsp.	6 tsp.	7 tsp.	8 tsp.	8 tsp.

Day/Date:

Breakfast: _____ Lunch: _____

Dinner: _____ Snack: _____

Group	Fruits	Vegetables	Grains	Meat & Beans	Milk	Oils
Goal Amount						
Estimate Your Total						
Increase ⇧ or Decrease? ⇩						

Physical Activity: _____ Spiritual Activity: _____

Steps/Miles/Minutes: _____

Day/Date:

Breakfast: _____ Lunch: _____

Dinner: _____ Snack: _____

Group	Fruits	Vegetables	Grains	Meat & Beans	Milk	Oils
Goal Amount						
Estimate Your Total						
Increase ⇧ or Decrease? ⇩						

Physical Activity: _____ Spiritual Activity: _____

Steps/Miles/Minutes: _____

Day/Date:

Breakfast: _____ Lunch: _____

Dinner: _____ Snack: _____

Group	Fruits	Vegetables	Grains	Meat & Beans	Milk	Oils
Goal Amount						
Estimate Your Total						
Increase ⇧ or Decrease? ⇩						

Physical Activity: _____ Spiritual Activity: _____

Steps/Miles/Minutes: _____

Day/Date:

Breakfast: _____   Lunch: _____
_____
Dinner: _____   Snack: _____
_____

Group	Fruits	Vegetables	Grains	Meat & Beans	Milk	Oils
Goal Amount						
Estimate Your Total						
Increase ⇧ or Decrease? ⇩						

Physical Activity: _____   Spiritual Activity: _____
Steps/Miles/Minutes: _____   _____

Day/Date:

Breakfast: _____   Lunch: _____
_____
Dinner: _____   Snack: _____
_____

Group	Fruits	Vegetables	Grains	Meat & Beans	Milk	Oils
Goal Amount						
Estimate Your Total						
Increase ⇧ or Decrease? ⇩						

Physical Activity: _____   Spiritual Activity: _____
Steps/Miles/Minutes: _____   _____

Day/Date:

Breakfast: _____   Lunch: _____
_____
Dinner: _____   Snack: _____
_____

Group	Fruits	Vegetables	Grains	Meat & Beans	Milk	Oils
Goal Amount						
Estimate Your Total						
Increase ⇧ or Decrease? ⇩						

Physical Activity: _____   Spiritual Activity: _____
Steps/Miles/Minutes: _____   _____

Day/Date:

Breakfast: _____   Lunch: _____
_____
Dinner: _____   Snack: _____
_____

Group	Fruits	Vegetables	Grains	Meat & Beans	Milk	Oils
Goal Amount						
Estimate Your Total						
Increase ⇧ or Decrease? ⇩						

Physical Activity: _____   Spiritual Activity: _____
Steps/Miles/Minutes: _____   _____

Live It Tracker

Name: _____ Loss/gain: _____ lbs.

Date: _____ Week #: ____ Calorie Range: _____ My food goal for next week: _____

Activity Level: None, < 30 min/day, 30-60 min/day, 60+ min/day My activity goal for next week: _____

Group	Daily Calories							
	1300-1400	1500-1600	1700-1800	1900-2000	2100-2200	2300-2400	2500-2600	2700-2800
Fruits	1.5-2 c.	1.5-2 c.	1.5-2 c.	2-2.5 c.	2-2.5 c.	2.5-3.5 c.	3.5-4.5 c.	3.5-4.5 c.
Vegetables	1.5-2 c.	2-2.5 c.	2.5-3 c.	2.5-3 c.	3-3.5 c.	3.5-4.5 c.	4.5-5 c.	4.5-5 c.
Grains	5 oz-eq.	5-6 oz-eq.	6-7 oz-eq.	6-7 oz-eq.	7-8 oz-eq.	8-9 oz-eq.	9-10 oz-eq.	10-11 oz-eq.
Meat & Beans	4 oz-eq.	5 oz-eq.	5-5.5 oz-eq.	5.5-6.5 oz-eq.	6.5-7 oz-eq.	7-7.5 oz-eq.	7-7.5 oz-eq.	7.5-8 oz-eq.
Milk	2-3 c.	3 c.	3 c.	3 c.	3 c.	3 c.	3 c.	3 c.
Healthy Oils	4 tsp.	5 tsp.	5 tsp.	6 tsp.	6 tsp.	7 tsp.	8 tsp.	8 tsp.

Day/Date: _____

Breakfast: _____ Lunch: _____

Dinner: _____ Snack: _____

Group	Fruits	Vegetables	Grains	Meat & Beans	Milk	Oils
Goal Amount						
Estimate Your Total						
Increase ⬆ or Decrease? ⬇						

Physical Activity: _____ Spiritual Activity: _____

Steps/Miles/Minutes: _____

Day/Date: _____

Breakfast: _____ Lunch: _____

Dinner: _____ Snack: _____

Group	Fruits	Vegetables	Grains	Meat & Beans	Milk	Oils
Goal Amount						
Estimate Your Total						
Increase ⬆ or Decrease? ⬇						

Physical Activity: _____ Spiritual Activity: _____

Steps/Miles/Minutes: _____

Day/Date: _____

Breakfast: _____ Lunch: _____

Dinner: _____ Snack: _____

Group	Fruits	Vegetables	Grains	Meat & Beans	Milk	Oils
Goal Amount						
Estimate Your Total						
Increase ⬆ or Decrease? ⬇						

Physical Activity: _____ Spiritual Activity: _____

Steps/Miles/Minutes: _____

Day/Date:

Breakfast: _____   Lunch: _____

Dinner: _____   Snack: _____

Group	Fruits	Vegetables	Grains	Meat & Beans	Milk	Oils
Goal Amount						
Estimate Your Total						
Increase ⬆ or Decrease? ⬇						

Physical Activity: _____   Spiritual Activity: _____

Steps/Miles/Minutes: _____   _____

Day/Date:

Breakfast: _____   Lunch: _____

Dinner: _____   Snack: _____

Group	Fruits	Vegetables	Grains	Meat & Beans	Milk	Oils
Goal Amount						
Estimate Your Total						
Increase ⬆ or Decrease? ⬇						

Physical Activity: _____   Spiritual Activity: _____

Steps/Miles/Minutes: _____   _____

Day/Date:

Breakfast: _____   Lunch: _____

Dinner: _____   Snack: _____

Group	Fruits	Vegetables	Grains	Meat & Beans	Milk	Oils
Goal Amount						
Estimate Your Total						
Increase ⬆ or Decrease? ⬇						

Physical Activity: _____   Spiritual Activity: _____

Steps/Miles/Minutes: _____   _____

Day/Date:

Breakfast: _____   Lunch: _____

Dinner: _____   Snack: _____

Group	Fruits	Vegetables	Grains	Meat & Beans	Milk	Oils
Goal Amount						
Estimate Your Total						
Increase ⬆ or Decrease? ⬇						

Physical Activity: _____   Spiritual Activity: _____

Steps/Miles/Minutes: _____   _____

Live It Tracker

Name: _____ Loss/gain: _____ lbs.

Date: _____ Week #: ____ Calorie Range: _____ My food goal for next week: _____

Activity Level: None, < 30 min/day, 30-60 min/day, 60+ min/day My activity goal for next week: _____

Group	Daily Calories							
	1300-1400	1500-1600	1700-1800	1900-2000	2100-2200	2300-2400	2500-2600	2700-2800
Fruits	1.5-2 c.	1.5-2 c.	1.5-2 c.	2-2.5 c.	2-2.5 c.	2.5-3.5 c.	3.5-4.5 c.	3.5-4.5 c.
Vegetables	1.5-2 c.	2-2.5 c.	2.5-3 c.	2.5-3 c.	3-3.5 c.	3.5-4.5 c.	4.5-5 c.	4.5-5 c.
Grains	5 oz-eq.	5-6 oz-eq.	6-7 oz-eq.	6-7 oz-eq.	7-8 oz-eq.	8-9 oz-eq.	9-10 oz-eq.	10-11 oz-eq.
Meat & Beans	4 oz-eq.	5 oz-eq.	5-5.5 oz-eq.	5.5-6.5 oz-eq.	6.5-7 oz-eq.	7-7.5 oz-eq.	7-7.5 oz-eq.	7.5-8 oz-eq.
Milk	2-3 c.	3 c.	3 c.	3 c.	3 c.	3 c.	3 c.	3 c.
Healthy Oils	4 tsp.	5 tsp.	5 tsp.	6 tsp.	6 tsp.	7 tsp.	8 tsp.	8 tsp.

Day/Date: _____

Breakfast: _____ Lunch: _____

Dinner: _____ Snack: _____

Group	Fruits	Vegetables	Grains	Meat & Beans	Milk	Oils
Goal Amount						
Estimate Your Total						
Increase ⇧ or Decrease? ⇩						

Physical Activity: _____ Spiritual Activity: _____

Steps/Miles/Minutes: _____ _____

Day/Date: _____

Breakfast: _____ Lunch: _____

Dinner: _____ Snack: _____

Group	Fruits	Vegetables	Grains	Meat & Beans	Milk	Oils
Goal Amount						
Estimate Your Total						
Increase ⇧ or Decrease? ⇩						

Physical Activity: _____ Spiritual Activity: _____

Steps/Miles/Minutes: _____ _____

Day/Date: _____

Breakfast: _____ Lunch: _____

Dinner: _____ Snack: _____

Group	Fruits	Vegetables	Grains	Meat & Beans	Milk	Oils
Goal Amount						
Estimate Your Total						
Increase ⇧ or Decrease? ⇩						

Physical Activity: _____ Spiritual Activity: _____

Steps/Miles/Minutes: _____ _____

Day/Date:

Breakfast: _____   Lunch: _____

Dinner: _____   Snack: _____

Group	Fruits	Vegetables	Grains	Meat & Beans	Milk	Oils
Goal Amount						
Estimate Your Total						
Increase ⬆ or Decrease? ⬇						

Physical Activity: _____   Spiritual Activity: _____

Steps/Miles/Minutes: _____   _____

Day/Date:

Breakfast: _____   Lunch: _____

Dinner: _____   Snack: _____

Group	Fruits	Vegetables	Grains	Meat & Beans	Milk	Oils
Goal Amount						
Estimate Your Total						
Increase ⬆ or Decrease? ⬇						

Physical Activity: _____   Spiritual Activity: _____

Steps/Miles/Minutes: _____   _____

Day/Date:

Breakfast: _____   Lunch: _____

Dinner: _____   Snack: _____

Group	Fruits	Vegetables	Grains	Meat & Beans	Milk	Oils
Goal Amount						
Estimate Your Total						
Increase ⬆ or Decrease? ⬇						

Physical Activity: _____   Spiritual Activity: _____

Steps/Miles/Minutes: _____   _____

Day/Date:

Breakfast: _____   Lunch: _____

Dinner: _____   Snack: _____

Group	Fruits	Vegetables	Grains	Meat & Beans	Milk	Oils
Goal Amount						
Estimate Your Total						
Increase ⬆ or Decrease? ⬇						

Physical Activity: _____   Spiritual Activity: _____

Steps/Miles/Minutes: _____   _____

Live It Tracker

Name: _____ Loss/gain: _____ lbs.

Date: _____ Week #: ____ Calorie Range: _____ My food goal for next week: _____

Activity Level: None, < 30 min/day, 30-60 min/day, 60+ min/day My activity goal for next week: _____

Group	Daily Calories							
	1300-1400	1500-1600	1700-1800	1900-2000	2100-2200	2300-2400	2500-2600	2700-2800
Fruits	1.5-2 c.	1.5-2 c.	1.5-2 c.	2-2.5 c.	2-2.5 c.	2.5-3.5 c.	3.5-4.5 c.	3.5-4.5 c.
Vegetables	1.5-2 c.	2-2.5 c.	2.5-3 c.	2.5-3 c.	3-3.5 c.	3.5-4.5 c.	4.5-5 c.	4.5-5 c.
Grains	5 oz-eq.	5-6 oz-eq.	6-7 oz-eq.	6-7 oz-eq.	7-8 oz-eq.	8-9 oz-eq.	9-10 oz-eq.	10-11 oz-eq.
Meat & Beans	4 oz-eq.	5 oz-eq.	5-5.5 oz-eq.	5.5-6.5 oz-eq.	6.5-7 oz-eq.	7-7.5 oz-eq.	7-7.5 oz-eq.	7.5-8 oz-eq.
Milk	2-3 c.	3 c.	3 c.	3 c.	3 c.	3 c.	3 c.	3 c.
Healthy Oils	4 tsp.	5 tsp.	5 tsp.	6 tsp.	6 tsp.	7 tsp.	8 tsp.	8 tsp.

Day/Date:

Breakfast: _____ Lunch: _____

Dinner: _____ Snack: _____

Group	Fruits	Vegetables	Grains	Meat & Beans	Milk	Oils
Goal Amount						
Estimate Your Total						
Increase ⇧ or Decrease? ⇩						

Physical Activity: _____ Spiritual Activity: _____

Steps/Miles/Minutes: _____

Day/Date:

Breakfast: _____ Lunch: _____

Dinner: _____ Snack: _____

Group	Fruits	Vegetables	Grains	Meat & Beans	Milk	Oils
Goal Amount						
Estimate Your Total						
Increase ⇧ or Decrease? ⇩						

Physical Activity: _____ Spiritual Activity: _____

Steps/Miles/Minutes: _____

Day/Date:

Breakfast: _____ Lunch: _____

Dinner: _____ Snack: _____

Group	Fruits	Vegetables	Grains	Meat & Beans	Milk	Oils
Goal Amount						
Estimate Your Total						
Increase ⇧ or Decrease? ⇩						

Physical Activity: _____ Spiritual Activity: _____

Steps/Miles/Minutes: _____

Day/Date:

Breakfast: _____ Lunch: _____

Dinner: _____ Snack: _____

Group	Fruits	Vegetables	Grains	Meat & Beans	Milk	Oils
Goal Amount						
Estimate Your Total						
Increase ⇧ or Decrease? ⇩						

Physical Activity: _____ Spiritual Activity: _____

Steps/Miles/Minutes: _____

Day/Date:

Breakfast: _____ Lunch: _____

Dinner: _____ Snack: _____

Group	Fruits	Vegetables	Grains	Meat & Beans	Milk	Oils
Goal Amount						
Estimate Your Total						
Increase ⇧ or Decrease? ⇩						

Physical Activity: _____ Spiritual Activity: _____

Steps/Miles/Minutes: _____

Day/Date:

Breakfast: _____ Lunch: _____

Dinner: _____ Snack: _____

Group	Fruits	Vegetables	Grains	Meat & Beans	Milk	Oils
Goal Amount						
Estimate Your Total						
Increase ⇧ or Decrease? ⇩						

Physical Activity: _____ Spiritual Activity: _____

Stcps/Miles/Minutes: _____

Day/Date:

Breakfast: _____ Lunch: _____

Dinner: _____ Snack: _____

Group	Fruits	Vegetables	Grains	Meat & Beans	Milk	Oils
Goal Amount						
Estimate Your Total						
Increase ⇧ or Decrease? ⇩						

Physical Activity: _____ Spiritual Activity: _____

Steps/Miles/Minutes: _____

Live It Tracker

Name: _____ Loss/gain: _____ lbs.

Date: _____ Week #: ____ Calorie Range: _____ My food goal for next week: _____

Activity Level: None, < 30 min/day, 30-60 min/day, 60+ min/day My activity goal for next week: _____

Group	Daily Calories							
	1300-1400	1500-1600	1700-1800	1900-2000	2100-2200	2300-2400	2500-2600	2700-2800
Fruits	1.5-2 c.	1.5-2 c.	1.5-2 c.	2-2.5 c.	2-2.5 c.	2.5-3.5 c.	3.5-4.5 c.	3.5-4.5 c.
Vegetables	1.5-2 c.	2-2.5 c.	2.5-3 c.	2.5-3 c.	3-3.5 c.	3.5-4.5 c.	4.5-5 c.	4.5-5 c.
Grains	5 oz-eq.	5-6 oz-eq.	6-7 oz-eq.	6-7 oz-eq.	7-8 oz-eq.	8-9 oz-eq.	9-10 oz-eq.	10-11 oz-eq.
Meat & Beans	4 oz-eq.	5 oz-eq.	5-5.5 oz-eq.	5.5-6.5 oz-eq.	6.5-7 oz-eq.	7-7.5 oz-eq.	7-7.5 oz-eq.	7.5-8 oz-eq.
Milk	2-3 c.	3 c.	3 c.	3 c.	3 c.	3 c.	3 c.	3 c.
Healthy Oils	4 tsp.	5 tsp.	5 tsp.	6 tsp.	6 tsp.	7 tsp.	8 tsp.	8 tsp.

Day/Date:

Breakfast: _____ Lunch: _____

Dinner: _____ Snack: _____

Group	Fruits	Vegetables	Grains	Meat & Beans	Milk	Oils
Goal Amount						
Estimate Your Total						
Increase ⇧ or Decrease? ⇩						

Physical Activity: _____ Spiritual Activity: _____

Steps/Miles/Minutes: _____

Day/Date:

Breakfast: _____ Lunch: _____

Dinner: _____ Snack: _____

Group	Fruits	Vegetables	Grains	Meat & Beans	Milk	Oils
Goal Amount						
Estimate Your Total						
Increase ⇧ or Decrease? ⇩						

Physical Activity: _____ Spiritual Activity: _____

Steps/Miles/Minutes: _____

Day/Date:

Breakfast: _____ Lunch: _____

Dinner: _____ Snack: _____

Group	Fruits	Vegetables	Grains	Meat & Beans	Milk	Oils
Goal Amount						
Estimate Your Total						
Increase ⇧ or Decrease? ⇩						

Physical Activity: _____ Spiritual Activity: _____

Steps/Miles/Minutes: _____

Day/Date:

Breakfast: _____ Lunch: _____

Dinner: _____ Snack: _____

Group	Fruits	Vegetables	Grains	Meat & Beans	Milk	Oils
Goal Amount						
Estimate Your Total						
Increase ⇧ or Decrease? ⇩						

Physical Activity: _____ Spiritual Activity: _____

Steps/Miles/Minutes: _____ _____

Day/Date:

Breakfast: _____ Lunch: _____

Dinner: _____ Snack: _____

Group	Fruits	Vegetables	Grains	Meat & Beans	Milk	Oils
Goal Amount						
Estimate Your Total						
Increase ⇧ or Decrease? ⇩						

Physical Activity: _____ Spiritual Activity: _____

Steps/Miles/Minutes: _____ _____

Day/Date:

Breakfast: _____ Lunch: _____

Dinner: _____ Snack: _____

Group	Fruits	Vegetables	Grains	Meat & Beans	Milk	Oils
Goal Amount						
Estimate Your Total						
Increase ⇧ or Decrease? ⇩						

Physical Activity: _____ Spiritual Activity: _____

Steps/Miles/Minutes: _____ _____

Day/Date:

Breakfast: _____ Lunch: _____

Dinner: _____ Snack: _____

Group	Fruits	Vegetables	Grains	Meat & Beans	Milk	Oils
Goal Amount						
Estimate Your Total						
Increase ⇧ or Decrease? ⇩						

Physical Activity: _____ Spiritual Activity: _____

Steps/Miles/Minutes: _____ _____

Live It Tracker

Name: _____ Loss/gain: _____ lbs.

Date: _____ Week #: _____ Calorie Range: _____ My food goal for next week: _____

Activity Level: None, < 30 min/day, 30-60 min/day, 60+ min/day My activity goal for next week: _____

Group	Daily Calories							
	1300-1400	1500-1600	1700-1800	1900-2000	2100-2200	2300-2400	2500-2600	2700-2800
Fruits	1.5-2 c.	1.5-2 c.	1.5-2 c.	2-2.5 c.	2-2.5 c.	2.5-3.5 c.	3.5-4.5 c.	3.5-4.5 c.
Vegetables	1.5-2 c.	2-2.5 c.	2.5-3 c.	2.5-3 c.	3-3.5 c.	3.5-4.5 c.	4.5-5 c.	4.5-5 c.
Grains	5 oz-eq.	5-6 oz-eq.	6-7 oz-eq.	6-7 oz-eq.	7-8 oz-eq.	8-9 oz-eq.	9-10 oz-eq.	10-11 oz-eq.
Meat & Beans	4 oz-eq.	5 oz-eq.	5-5.5 oz-eq.	5.5-6.5 oz-eq.	6.5-7 oz-eq.	7-7.5 oz-eq.	7-7.5 oz-eq.	7.5-8 oz-eq.
Milk	2-3 c.	3 c.	3 c.	3 c.	3 c.	3 c.	3 c.	3 c.
Healthy Oils	4 tsp.	5 tsp.	5 tsp.	6 tsp.	6 tsp.	7 tsp.	8 tsp.	8 tsp.

Day/Date:

Breakfast: _____   Lunch: _____

Dinner: _____   Snack: _____

Group	Fruits	Vegetables	Grains	Meat & Beans	Milk	Oils
Goal Amount						
Estimate Your Total						
Increase ⇧ or Decrease? ⇩						

Physical Activity: _____   Spiritual Activity: _____

Steps/Miles/Minutes: _____

Day/Date:

Breakfast: _____   Lunch: _____

Dinner: _____   Snack: _____

Group	Fruits	Vegetables	Grains	Meat & Beans	Milk	Oils
Goal Amount						
Estimate Your Total						
Increase ⇧ or Decrease? ⇩						

Physical Activity: _____   Spiritual Activity: _____

Steps/Miles/Minutes: _____

Day/Date:

Breakfast: _____   Lunch: _____

Dinner: _____   Snack: _____

Group	Fruits	Vegetables	Grains	Meat & Beans	Milk	Oils
Goal Amount						
Estimate Your Total						
Increase ⇧ or Decrease? ⇩						

Physical Activity: _____   Spiritual Activity: _____

Steps/Miles/Minutes: _____

Day/Date: _____

Breakfast: _____ Lunch: _____

Dinner: _____ Snack: _____

Group	Fruits	Vegetables	Grains	Meat & Beans	Milk	Oils
Goal Amount						
Estimate Your Total						
Increase ⬆ or Decrease? ⬇						

Physical Activity: _____ Spiritual Activity: _____

Steps/Miles/Minutes: _____

Day/Date: _____

Breakfast: _____ Lunch: _____

Dinner: _____ Snack: _____

Group	Fruits	Vegetables	Grains	Meat & Beans	Milk	Oils
Goal Amount						
Estimate Your Total						
Increase ⬆ or Decrease? ⬇						

Physical Activity: _____ Spiritual Activity: _____

Steps/Miles/Minutes: _____

Day/Date: _____

Breakfast: _____ Lunch: _____

Dinner: _____ Snack: _____

Group	Fruits	Vegetables	Grains	Meat & Beans	Milk	Oils
Goal Amount						
Estimate Your Total						
Increase ⬆ or Decrease? ⬇						

Physical Activity: _____ Spiritual Activity: _____

Steps/Miles/Minutes: _____

Day/Date: _____

Breakfast: _____ Lunch: _____

Dinner: _____ Snack: _____

Group	Fruits	Vegetables	Grains	Meat & Beans	Milk	Oils
Goal Amount						
Estimate Your Total						
Increase ⬆ or Decrease? ⬇						

Physical Activity: _____ Spiritual Activity: _____

Steps/Miles/Minutes: _____

Live It Tracker

Name: _____ Loss/gain: _____ lbs.

Date: _____ Week #: ____ Calorie Range: _____ My food goal for next week: _____

Activity Level: None, < 30 min/day, 30-60 min/day, 60+ min/day My activity goal for next week: _____

Group	Daily Calories							
	1300-1400	1500-1600	1700-1800	1900-2000	2100-2200	2300-2400	2500-2600	2700-2800
Fruits	1.5-2 c.	1.5-2 c.	1.5-2 c.	2-2.5 c.	2-2.5 c.	2.5-3.5 c.	3.5-4.5 c.	3.5-4.5 c.
Vegetables	1.5-2 c.	2-2.5 c.	2.5-3 c.	2.5-3 c.	3-3.5 c.	3.5-4.5 c.	4.5-5 c.	4.5-5 c.
Grains	5 oz-eq.	5-6 oz-eq.	6-7 oz-eq.	6-7 oz-eq.	7-8 oz-eq.	8-9 oz-eq.	9-10 oz-eq.	10-11 oz-eq.
Meat & Beans	4 oz-eq.	5 oz-eq.	5-5.5 oz-eq.	5.5-6.5 oz-eq.	6.5-7 oz-eq.	7-7.5 oz-eq.	7-7.5 oz-eq.	7.5-8 oz-eq.
Milk	2-3 c.	3 c.	3 c.	3 c.	3 c.	3 c.	3 c.	3 c.
Healthy Oils	4 tsp.	5 tsp.	5 tsp.	6 tsp.	6 tsp.	7 tsp.	8 tsp.	8 tsp.

Day/Date: _____

Breakfast: _____   Lunch: _____

Dinner: _____   Snack: _____

Group	Fruits	Vegetables	Grains	Meat & Beans	Milk	Oils
Goal Amount						
Estimate Your Total						
Increase ⇧ or Decrease? ⇩						

Physical Activity: _____   Spiritual Activity: _____

Steps/Miles/Minutes: _____

Day/Date: _____

Breakfast: _____   Lunch: _____

Dinner: _____   Snack: _____

Group	Fruits	Vegetables	Grains	Meat & Beans	Milk	Oils
Goal Amount						
Estimate Your Total						
Increase ⇧ or Decrease? ⇩						

Physical Activity: _____   Spiritual Activity: _____

Steps/Miles/Minutes: _____

Day/Date: _____

Breakfast: _____   Lunch: _____

Dinner: _____   Snack: _____

Group	Fruits	Vegetables	Grains	Meat & Beans	Milk	Oils
Goal Amount						
Estimate Your Total						
Increase ⇧ or Decrease? ⇩						

Physical Activity: _____   Spiritual Activity: _____

Steps/Miles/Minutes: _____

Day/Date: _____

Breakfast: _____   Lunch: _____

Dinner: _____   Snack: _____

Group	Fruits	Vegetables	Grains	Meat & Beans	Milk	Oils
Goal Amount						
Estimate Your Total						
Increase ⇧ or Decrease? ⇩						

Physical Activity: _____   Spiritual Activity: _____

Steps/Miles/Minutes: _____   _____

Day/Date: _____

Breakfast: _____   Lunch: _____

Dinner: _____   Snack: _____

Group	Fruits	Vegetables	Grains	Meat & Beans	Milk	Oils
Goal Amount						
Estimate Your Total						
Increase ⇧ or Decrease? ⇩						

Physical Activity: _____   Spiritual Activity: _____

Steps/Miles/Minutes: _____   _____

Day/Date: _____

Breakfast: _____   Lunch: _____

Dinner: _____   Snack: _____

Group	Fruits	Vegetables	Grains	Meat & Beans	Milk	Oils
Goal Amount						
Estimate Your Total						
Increase ⇧ or Decrease? ⇩						

Physical Activity: _____   Spiritual Activity: _____

Steps/Miles/Minutes: _____   _____

Day/Date: _____

Breakfast: _____   Lunch: _____

Dinner: _____   Snack: _____

Group	Fruits	Vegetables	Grains	Meat & Beans	Milk	Oils
Goal Amount						
Estimate Your Total						
Increase ⇧ or Decrease? ⇩						

Physical Activity: _____   Spiritual Activity: _____

Steps/Miles/Minutes: _____   _____

let's count our miles!

Join the 100-Mile Club this Session

Can't walk that mile yet? Don't be discouraged! There are exercises you can do to strengthen your body and burn those extra calories. Keep a record on your Live It Tracker of the number of minutes you do these common physical activities, convert those minutes to miles following the chart below, and then mark off each mile you have completed on the chart found on the back of the front cover. Report your miles to your 100-Mile Club representative when you first arrive each week. Remember, you are not competing with anyone else . . . just yourself. Your job is to strive to reach 100 miles before the last meeting in this session. You can do it—just keep on moving!

Walking
slowly, 2 mph	30 min. = 156 cal. = 1 mile
moderately, 3 mph	20 min. = 156 cal. = 1 mile
very briskly, 4 mph	15 min. = 156 cal. = 1 mile
speed walking	10 min. = 156 cal. = 1 mile
up stairs	13 min. = 159 cal. = 1 mile

Running/Jogging
10 min. = 156 cal. = 1 mile

Cycling Outdoors
slowly, <10 mph	20 min. = 156 cal. = 1 mile
light effort, 10-12 mph	12 min. = 156 cal. = 1 mile
moderate effort, 12-14 mph	10 min. = 156 cal. = 1 mile
vigorous effort, 14-16 mph	7.5 min. = 156 cal. = 1 mile
very fast, 16-19 mph	6.5 min. = 152 cal. = 1 mile

Sports Activities
Playing tennis (singles)	10 min. = 156 cal. = 1 mile
Swimming	
light to moderate effort	11 min. = 152 cal. = 1 mile
fast, vigorous effort	7.5 min. = 156 cal. = 1 mile
Softball	15 min. = 156 cal. = 1 mile
Golf	20 min. = 156 cal = 1 mile
Rollerblading	6.5 min. = 152 cal. = 1 mile
Ice skating	11 min. = 152 cal. = 1 mile

Jumping rope	7.5 min. = 156 cal. = 1 mile
Basketball	12 min. = 156 cal. = 1 mile
Soccer (casual)	15 min. = 159 cal. = 1 mile

Around the House

Mowing grass	22 min. = 156 cal. = 1 mile
Mopping, sweeping, vacuuming	19.5 min. = 155 cal. = 1 mile
Cooking	40 min. =160 cal. = 1 mile
Gardening	19 min. = 156 cal. = 1 mile
Housework (general)	35 min. = 156 cal. = 1 mile
Ironing	45 min. = 153 cal. = 1 mile
Raking leaves	25 min. = 150 cal. = 1 mile
Washing car	23 min. = 156 cal. = 1 mile
Washing dishes	45 min. = 153 cal. = 1 mile

At the Gym

Stair machine	8.5 min. = 155 cal. = 1 mile
Stationary bike	
slowly, 10 mph	30 min. = 156 cal. = 1 mile
moderately, 10-13 mph	15 min. = 156 cal. = 1 mile
vigorously, 13-16 mph	7.5 min. = 156 cal. = 1 mile
briskly, 16-19 mph	6.5 min. = 156 cal. = 1 mile
Elliptical trainer	12 min. = 156 cal. = 1 mile
Weight machines (used vigorously)	13 min. = 152 cal.=1 mile
Aerobics	
low impact	15 min. = 156 cal. = 1 mile
high impact	12 min. = 156 cal. = 1 mile
water	20 min. = 156 cal. = 1 mile
Pilates	15 min. = 156 cal. = 1 mile
Raquetball (casual)	15 min. = 159 cal. = 1 mile
Stretching exercises	25 min. = 150 cal. = 1 mile
Weight lifting (also works for weight machines used moderately or gently)	30 min. = 156 cal. = 1 mile

Family Leisure

Playing piano	37 min. = 155 cal. = 1 mile
Jumping rope	10 min. = 152 cal. = 1 mile
Skating (moderate)	20 min. = 152 cal. = 1 mile
Swimming	
moderate	17 min. = 156 cal. = 1 mile
vigorous	10 min. = 148 cal. = 1 mile
Table tennis	25 min. = 150 cal. = 1 mile
Walk/run/play with kids	25 min. = 150 cal. = 1 mile

The Power of Hope

Balanced Living
Scripture Memory Verses:

Proverbs 13:12

Psalm 42:5-6

Colossians 1:13-14

Romans 12:12

Hebrews 11:1

Psalm 62:5

Luke 6:46

Hebrews 10:23

Romans 5:5

Psalm 71:14

Week 2: Heartsick and Battle Weary

*Hope deferred makes the heart sick,
But a longing fulfilled is a tree of life.*

Week 3: Put Your Hope in God

*Why are you downcast, O my soul?
Why so disturbed within me?
Put your hope in God, for I will yet
praise him, my Savior and my God.*

HOW TO USE THESE CARDS:

Separate cards from the Bible study book. These cards are designed to be used when exercising. To do this, you may want to punch a hole in the upper left corner of the cards and place on a ring. When you have finished memorizing all the verses from one study, add the new Bible study cards to the ring and continue practicing the old verses while learning the new ones. Cards may be placed anywhere you will see them regularly—on the dashboard of your car, on a mirror, on a desk. After you have memorized the verse, begin using the reverse side of the card so the reference is connected to the verse. This is a great way to practice the verses you have already learned.

PROVERBS 13:12

PSALM 42:5-6

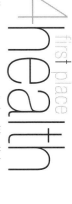

4 first place health

discover a new way to healthy living

Week 6: Faith Ensures Hope

Now faith is being sure of what we hope for and certain of what we do not see.

Week 7: Knowledge Increases Hope

Find rest, O my soul, in God alone; my hope comes from him.

Week 4: Forgiveness Renews Hope

He has rescued us from the dominion of darkness and brought us into the kingdom of the Son he loves, in whom we have redemption, the forgiveness of sins.

Week 5: Hope Leads to Action

Be joyful in hope, patient in affliction, faithful in prayer.

HEBREWS 11:1

COLOSSIANS 1:13-14

PSALM 62:5

ROMANS 12:12

Week 10: Hope Does Not Disappoint

And hope does not disappoint us, because God has poured out his love into our hearts by the Holy Spirit, whom he has given us.

Week 11: Overflowing Hope

But as for me, I will always have hope; I will praise you more and more.

Week 8: Obedience Builds Hope

Why do you call me "Lord, Lord," and do not do what I say?

Week 9: Hope Perseveres

Let us hold unswervingly to the hope we possess, for he who promised is faithful.

ROMANS 5:5

LUKE 6:46

PSALM 71:14

HEBREWS 10:23